Praise for *Diabetes Type 2: Complete Food Management Program*

"This is a comprehensive and pertinent guide to successful diabetes management. It offers practical solutions to a complex problem. With obesity and its related health problems on the rise in the United States, this provides a valuable resource to help us all pay attention to the lifestyle and food choices we make everyday. I highly recommend it."

—**Marlene Bedrich, R.N., C.D.E., program coordinator, Diabetes Teaching Center, University of California San Francisco Medical Center**

"A comprehensive, easy-to-read resource to assist people with type 2 diabetes on how to incorporate nutrition therapy into their diabetes management. The book provides practical information on nutrition therapy that can be put to use right away. Nutrition therapy, an essential part of diabetes care, is often a piece on which people with diabetes receive little information. The invaluable information in this guide will help empower people with type 2 diabetes to engage in self-care of their diabetes."

—**Lisa Kroon, Pharm.D., C.D.E, assistant clinical professor of pharmacy, University of California San Francisco, School of Pharmacy**

"An excellent reference for patients as well as a valuable resource for myself as a clinician caring for patients with type 2 diabetes."

—**Carolyn Muir, R.N., M.S., N.P., nurse practitioner**

"I am very impressed with this book. It is a comprehensive, thorough resource, packed with practical information. It is informative and current, and while focused on nutrition, nicely links these principles to important questions regarding exercise and drug therapies, among other issues. The text is user-friendly and is written in a manner that is easy to understand. I would recommend it to all my patients with diabetes, type 2 or type 1."

—**Stephen M. Rosenthal, M.D., professor of pediatrics, University of California San Francisco**

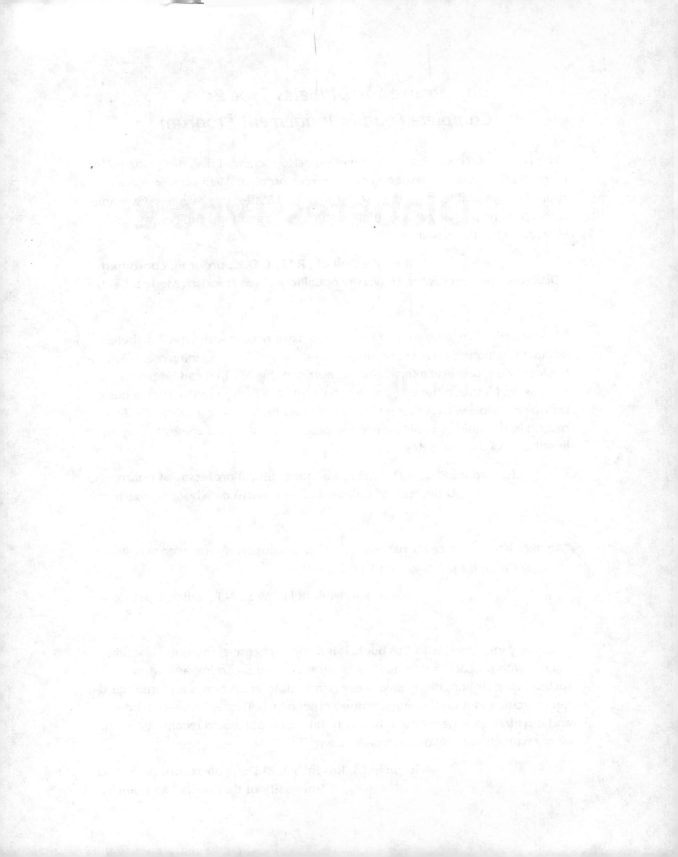

Diabetes Type 2: Complete Food Management Program

Sherri Shafer, R.D., C.D.E.

PRIMA PUBLISHING

Published by Prima Publishing, Roseville, California. Member of the Crown Publishing Group, a division of Random House, Inc.

PRIMA PUBLISHING and colophon are trademarks of Random House, Inc., registered with the United States Patent and Trademark Office.

This book is intended only as a starting point for gathering information on diabetes. As with all matters concerning one's health, the reader should consult with a doctor before embarking on any health program.

Illustrations on pages 34, 36, 54, 145, and 175 courtesy of Michael Flodquist.
Illustrations on pages 25, 26, 35, 70, 71, 72, 74, and 121 courtesy of Paula Gray.

Library of Congress Cataloging-in-Publication Data
    Shafer, Sherri.
        Diabetes type 2: complete food management program / Sherri Shafer
        p.   cm.
    Includes index.
    ISBN 0-7615-3252-8
    1. Non-insulin-dependent diabetes—Diet therapy. I. Title: Diabetes type two.
    II. Title.
    RC662.181.553   2001
    616.41620654—dc21   200151346

02 03 04 05 DD 10 9 8 7 6 5 4 3 2
Printed in the United States of America

First Edition

Visit us online at www.primapublishing.com

To my husband, Richard, and my son, Carter. I'm so fortunate to have you both.
You've brought me the most precious days of my life.

Contents

- Lowfat on the go (fast food, airlines)
- Reducing cholesterol intake
- Reducing sodium intake
  - Shopping low-sodium
  - Low-sodium cooking
  - Low-sodium restaurant tips
- Reducing sugar intake
- Strategies for special occasions and holidays

Acknowledgments

The opportunity to write this book presented itself shortly after the birth of my son. Luckily, I had a remarkably happy and content baby. My husband, Richard, provided encouragement and made room in our lives for me to write. I appreciate every day we've had together, and anticipate the days we have yet to share.

I'd like to thank Jamie Miller and Andrew Vallas, and the rest of the dedicated staff at Prima, for bringing this project to fruition.

My parents, Ron and Jan, and my siblings, Cindy, Michael, and Pat, have provided lifelong love and support.

I've been blessed with many wonderful friends who have kept me laughing, given me perspective, and have always been there when I've needed them.

I'm indebted to my mentors and coworkers at UCSF Medical Center for providing so much opportunity for professional growth and learning.

I especially want to thank the many people with diabetes who have touched my life, and have allowed me to touch their lives in return.

Introduction: Dealing with the Diagnosis

You may be newly diagnosed or you may have known about your diabetes for some time. Either way, you probably remember the day that you received the diagnosis. Maybe you halfway expected it, because it runs in your family. Or maybe the diagnosis took you by complete surprise and threw your life into a tailspin. Your initial response may have been denial, depression, anger, or fear. It's not uncommon to go through a whole series of emotions when confronted with any chronic illness. It's important to allow yourself to feel those emotions. Working through difficult feelings can lead you down the path to acceptance. Once acceptance settles in, then you're on firm ground. You can care for your diabetes and get on with enjoying your life.

The thought of diabetes may conjure up some pretty scary images if you've known someone who suffered from diabetes-related complications. It's true that uncontrolled diabetes can lead to serious health problems. Fortunately, the last couple of decades have brought remarkable advancements in the field of diabetes care. Reams of scientific reports and study findings have taught us how to best treat diabetes. Nutritional management strategies and the importance of exercise are now well understood. There has been an explosion of technological advances in the realm of home blood-sugar monitoring. Many new medications have been created that can successfully treat diabetes. Unfortunately, some people developed diabetes before such good treatment options existed. In addition, certain people haven't had access to good health care or diabetes education. In this day and age, you can do much to prevent diabetes-related health problems and live a healthy and happy life. *Diabetes doesn't automatically cause complications, but uncontrolled diabetes can lead to them.* Let's try to make diabetes complications a thing of the past!

One of the most important studies ever done in relation to type 2 diabetes, was the United Kingdom Prospective Diabetes Study (UKPDS). The UKPDS enrolled 5,102 people with newly diagnosed type 2 diabetes and monitored their blood sugar and blood pressure treatments for approximately 10 years. Significant findings showed that for every percentage point decrease in the hemoglobin A1c (HbA1c), there was a 25 percent reduction in diabetes-related deaths and an 18 percent reduction in heart attacks. (HbA1c is a test that measures blood sugar control over the previous few months.) Lowering blood pressure reduced the incidence of strokes by 44 percent, heart failure by 56 percent, deterioration of vision by 47 percent, diabetes-related deaths by 32 percent, and diseases of the eyes and kidneys by 37 percent. Achieving control was the goal, whether by diet therapy alone or through the use of combined medications. The take-home message of the UKPDS is that *both blood sugar control and blood pressure control* greatly reduce the complications associated with diabetes.

Another landmark study was the Diabetes Control and Complications Trial (DCCT). This was a 10-year study to find out if blood sugar control delayed or prevented diabetes-related complications. The DCCT enrolled 1,441 people with type 1 diabetes. Individuals were separated into two study groups. Members of one group received intensive education and treatment to control their diabetes. The other group received a more conventional, less stringent management approach. The intensively managed group had better blood sugar control. As a result, participants had on average, a 76 percent reduction in retinopathy (eye damage), a 60 percent reduction in neuropathy (nerve damage), and a 54 percent reduction in albuminuria. (Albuminuria reflects kidney damage.)

Diabetes is a controllable disease. To control diabetes, you must first learn about the disease and how it is managed. Knowledge is an important key to controlling diabetes and maintaining health and well-being. Diet modifications and exercise are the first line of defense in managing type 2 diabetes. If blood sugar levels aren't maintained within target ranges by those primary interventions, then medication should be added. Some individuals need medication no matter how carefully they eat and exercise. Whether or not you'll need medication depends upon many factors and can be assessed by your health-care provider.

Learn everything that you can about diabetes and its treatment. Seek evaluation and treatment from health-care professionals who understand the intricacies of diabetes management. Take what you learn and use it to manage your diabetes now and throughout your future.

CHAPTER 1

Diabetes Defined

❦

IN THIS CHAPTER

- The different types of diabetes
- The signs and symptoms of diabetes
- How diabetes is diagnosed
- Complications

This book focuses on the nutritional management of diabetes. Before we begin, however, I think it's important to provide some general information about the disease.

Diabetes mellitus is a disorder that results in elevated blood sugar levels. Having some sugar in the blood is normal. In fact, it's necessary. The sugar in the blood is called glucose. Glucose is the fuel that makes the brain work, the heart contract, and the muscles move. It nourishes and fuels all of the tissues in the body. Carbohydrate foods provide the glucose that we need, and digestion makes the glucose from the food available to be absorbed into the bloodstream. The network of blood vessels transports this vital sugar throughout the body to the awaiting tissues, muscles, and cells. An organ called the pancreas (nestled in next to the stomach) makes a hormone called insulin. Insulin helps to shuttle the glucose into the cells and is required for proper use and storage of proteins and fats. In the case of diabetes, there is a defect with the insulin—either the pancreas is not making insulin (type 1 diabetes), or the insulin isn't working properly to shuttle glucose into the cells (type 2 diabetes). Diabetes results when there is an imbalance between glucose and insulin, and blood sugar levels rise above the normal range. (Note: The terms blood glucose and blood sugar are used interchangeably in this book.)

History reveals written descriptions of the disease that date back as far as 1500 B.C. Records describe a disorder characterized by increased urination and thirst. The word *diabetes* comes from a Greek term meaning "to flow through," which described the passage of water through the body. The word *mellitus* comes from the Latin term for "honey." It described the quality of the urine. The urine was sweet because sugar was being passed in the urine. If you were a doctor back in those days, you had the privilege of tasting the urine to make the diagnosis—they didn't have any laboratory tests or blood sugar meters!

Approximately 16 million Americans—almost 7 percent of the country's population—have diabetes. Most of them have type 2 diabetes. At least one-third of the people with type 2 diabetes don't even know that they have the disease yet! It has become an epidemic. Why? Because, as a population, we are gaining too much weight and are exercising less. Obesity and inactivity are major risk factors for getting type 2 diabetes.

> At least one-third of the people with type 2 diabetes don't even know that they have the disease yet.

Type 2 diabetes is on the rise, with approximately 800,000 new cases each year. Also alarming is that type 2 diabetes now strikes at younger ages than ever before. Even children and teens are being diagnosed with type 2 diabetes, the kind of diabetes that was once referred to as "adult onset diabetes."

Left untreated, diabetes can lead to many different complications. In the United States, diabetes is still the leading cause of blindness, end-stage kidney disease, and amputation. But there is no reason to let diabetes go untreated. Proper treatment can greatly reduce the risk of suffering ill effects from the disease. Arm yourself with knowledge. Learn about your diabetes and how to best take care of it.

The Different Types of Diabetes

Type 1 diabetes is caused by destruction of the cells that make insulin. The beta cells of the pancreas, which normally make insulin, are destroyed by the body's own immune cells. Immune cells are supposed to destroy invading viruses and bacteria. These fighter cells mistakenly destroy the cells that produce insulin. Because insulin is necessary for life, people with type 1 diabetes must take daily insulin injections to survive.

Type 1 diabetes is often referred to as insulin-dependent diabetes mellitus, which may be abbreviated as IDDM. It was once known as juvenile diabetes, or childhood-onset diabetes. However, as it is not uncommon for people to first get this type of diabetes when they are adults, the preferred term is "type 1 diabetes."

The predisposition for developing type 1 diabetes is inherited. Only about 5–10 percent of all cases of diabetes are type 1.

Type 2 diabetes is the most common form of diabetes. About 90–95 percent of all cases of diabetes are type 2. A strong genetic component exists in type 2 diabetes—meaning it runs in families—so screening is important for anyone at increased risk. It is estimated that on average, most people have had type 2 diabetes for at least six full years before it was actually diagnosed!

Type 2 diabetes is also known as non-insulin dependent diabetes, which may be abbreviated NIDDM. Yet as many as 40 percent of people with type 2 diabetes do use injected insulin to help control their blood sugar, so the preferred term is "type 2 diabetes." Type 2 diabetes used to be called adult-onset diabetes; however, more and more children and teens are getting this form of the disease. High-fat diets and sedentary lifestyles have caused an alarming increase in childhood obesity, which has contributed to type 2 diabetes striking our young.

Insulin resistance characterizes this type of diabetes. That means that the body has insulin, but the insulin doesn't work well. Insulin is supposed to act like a key to unlock the body's cells, allowing glucose to move into the cells where it is needed for fuel. In the case of type 2 diabetes, the cells are not sensitive to the insulin. The key doesn't open the door properly, and the glucose backs up in the blood, resulting in high blood sugar. Oftentimes the pancreas tries to compensate by making more insulin. This can wear the pancreas down, and, eventually, it may no longer be able to produce adequate amounts of insulin. Type 2 diabetes is marked by defects in insulin action, insulin production, or both.

Another defect associated with type 2 diabetes is the excess output of sugar from the liver. The liver plays an important role in normal glucose regulation by providing a storage site for extra glucose that isn't immediately needed after the meal. Extra mealtime glucose is stored in the liver and in the muscles. The storage form of glucose is called glycogen. Hours after mealtime, the body may need more fuel, and thus more glucose. The liver then breaks down the stored glycogen and releases the needed glucose into the bloodstream. When glucose is really at a shortage, the liver can make a certain amount of brand new glucose. Sometimes, with type 2 diabetes, the liver doesn't regulate glucose properly. The liver may release too much sugar even when the body doesn't need it. That's why your blood sugar may be high in the morning before you've had anything to eat.

Obesity and physical inactivity both cause insulin resistance. As many as three out of every four people with type 2 diabetes are overweight. Weight loss, proper diet, and regular exercise are all important in preventing and treating type 2 diabetes.

Risk factors for type 2 diabetes:

- Family history: someone in your family has type 2 diabetes
- Obesity: BMI of 27 or higher (see chapter 4 for more on BMI)
- Age: greater than 45 (but, remember, type 2 diabetes can strike younger people as well)
- Ethnicity (African Americans, Hispanic Americans, Native Americans, Asian Americans, and Pacific Islanders)
- High blood pressure

- High triglycerides (blood fats)

- High cholesterol

- Low levels of HDL (too little of the "good" type of cholesterol)

- Lack of physical activity

- Previous history of abnormal blood sugar levels (impaired glucose tolerance)

- Polycystic ovary syndrome

- Previous history of gestational diabetes

- Previous history of delivering a baby weighing over nine pounds

Anyone who has any of the previous risk factors should be screened for type 2 diabetes right away, and if negative, should be rescreened at least every three years. For individuals without known risk factors, screening should begin at age 45 and be repeated every three years.

Gestational diabetes mellitus (abbreviated GDM) is also known as diabetes in pregnancy. Pregnancy hormones increase the demand for insulin. Normally, the expectant mother's pancreas will step up the insulin production to meet those demands. However, in about 7 percent of all pregnancies, the woman's pancreas cannot produce enough insulin to keep her blood sugar controlled. The result is high blood sugar, which usually develops during the latter half of the pregnancy. Women are routinely tested for this condition between 24 and 28 weeks of pregnancy. (A normal pregnancy lasts 40 weeks.)

> It is estimated that on average, most people have had type 2 diabetes for at least six full years before it was actually diagnosed.

The screening test involves drinking a sugary beverage that contains 50 grams of glucose and having the blood sugar tested one hour later. A normal value is below 140 mg/dl (milligrams per deciliter). If the blood sugar level is 140 mg/dl or higher, an oral glucose tolerance test (OGTT) is usually performed. A sugary beverage containing 100 grams of glucose is consumed after an overnight fast.

The blood sugar is tested before the drink is consumed, and then again at one-hour intervals for the next three hours. (To convert mg/dl [milligrams per deciliter] to mmol/l [millimoles per liter], divide by 18.)

Normal values for the OGTT are as follows:

Fasting: below 95 mg/dl

One hour: below 180 mg/dl

Two hours: below 155 mg/dl

Three hours: below 140 mg/dl

Having GDM classifies the pregnancy as high-risk, requiring stringent blood sugar control to reduce possible harm to the fetus and help assure a safe delivery. Prenatal care and close monitoring are extremely important. Dietary modifications are the main treatment for GDM, though if blood glucose levels cannot be maintained in the normal range, insulin injections are added. Diabetes pills are not recommended during pregnancy. Once the baby is delivered, there is a shift in maternal hormones, and the demand for insulin returns to normal. The woman's pancreas can keep up again, and the gestational diabetes is gone. It is important to monitor the blood sugar after delivery to confirm that the diabetes is gone. If the blood sugar remains elevated, the diabetes may be reclassified as type 2 diabetes.

> Blood sugar monitoring is an important tool in achieving control.

If you've had gestational diabetes in one pregnancy, you're likely to have it again in future pregnancies, and any woman who has had GDM has a significant chance of developing type 2 diabetes sometime later in life. The best prevention is maintaining a near-normal weight and exercising regularly. Any woman who has had GDM should be screened at least every 3 years for the onset of type 2 diabetes.

Tip: If you've had GDM in a previous pregnancy, get screened *before* becoming pregnant again, since as many as 40–60 percent of women with GDM eventually get type 2 diabetes. Undiagnosed type 2 diabetes can cause serious problems to the developing fetus.

Tip: When women with a previous history of GDM get pregnant again, they should be screened for GDM earlier in their pregnancies, prior to 24 weeks of gestation.

Risk factors for gestational diabetes mellitus (GDM) include:

• Obesity

• Family history of diabetes

• History of glucose intolerance (a history of blood sugar above normal range)

• Taking medications that cause glucose intolerance

• Age over 25

• The following ethnic groups: African American, Hispanic American, Asian American, Native American, and Pacific Islanders

Tip: Women who fit the previous criteria should be screened for GDM at their first prenatal visit. If the test is negative, they should be retested between 24 and 28 weeks of gestation.

For more information on diabetes during pregnancy, see chapter 14.

Other causes of diabetes: Diseases that affect the pancreas such as cystic fibrosis, pancreatitis, and hemochromatosis can lead to abnormal insulin production and diabetes. Injury to the pancreas can also disrupt normal insulin production. Also, various drugs and steroids, including prednisone, can lead to insulin resistance, which may result in elevated blood sugar.

The Signs and Symptoms of Diabetes

Frequent urination: High blood sugar causes increased urination as the body tries to get rid of the sugar via the urine.

Thirst: Excessive urination can lead to dehydration. Thirst is a natural response to assure fluid replacement.

Hunger: If the sugar accumulates in the bloodstream instead of getting into the cells where it is needed, the cells aren't being fed and that can trigger hunger.

Blurred vision: When the blood sugar goes too high, the lenses of the eyes absorb extra sugar and water, which can temporarily distort the shape of the lenses. This leads to blurred vision. When blood sugar levels return to normal, the shape of the lenses returns to normal and the blurred vision resolves.

Some people don't realize that they have diabetes and the blurred vision causes them to get new glasses. Then when they get control of their diabetes, their vision returns to what it once was and the glasses are useless.

Tip: Don't get new eyeglasses when your blood sugar is out of control. Wait until your blood sugar is well managed before you obtain new eyeglasses.

> Anyone who has risk factors should be screened for type 2 diabetes right away, and if negative, should be rescreened at least every three years.

Fatigue: High blood sugar can make you feel tired, heavy, or lethargic.

Urinary tract infections and skin infections: High sugar creates a sweet environment. Bacteria can thrive in a sweet environment.

Yeast infections: High sugar creates a sweet environment, which can lead to overgrowth of yeast.

Weight loss: Weight loss can occur because the sugar is accumulating in the blood instead of nourishing the cells as it should. The kidneys are dumping sugar into the urine, and those calories are being flushed down the toilet. This is not a healthful way to lose weight! High blood sugar, if left untreated, can lead to complications.

Note: Many people with type 2 diabetes have no symptoms whatsoever. That's why it's so important to find out if you have diabetes, and to obtain treatment if you do.

How Diabetes Is Diagnosed

The blood sugar can be tested in a fasting state (which means no food or calories have been consumed for at least 8 hours), or it can be tested randomly without concern for what has been eaten. (The preferred screening test is the fasting test.) The value will either be normal (non-diabetic) or abnormal. If it is slightly elevated, the category is called impaired glucose tolerance (IGT), which just means that the number is above normal but not yet high enough to be classified as diabetes. (Values are listed in milligrams per deciliter [mg/dl]. If you are more familiar with numbers that are listed in millimoles per liter [mmol/l], you can convert mg/dl to mmol/l by dividing by 18.)

> Approximately 16 million Americans—almost 7 percent of the country's population—have diabetes. Most of them have type 2 diabetes.

Fasting Blood Glucose (No Food for 8 Hours)

Normal is less than 110 mg/dl.

Impaired glucose tolerance is 110 to 125 mg/dl.

Diabetes diagnosis is 126 mg/dl or higher.

Random Blood Glucose (Taken 1–2 Hours After Eating)

Normal is less than 140 mg/dl.

Impaired glucose tolerance is 140 to 199 mg/dl.

Diabetes diagnosis is 200 or above, and symptoms of diabetes are present.

To confirm a diagnosis of diabetes, the blood test is repeated on a separate occasion. Another test called the oral glucose tolerance test (OGTT) may be prescribed to be certain of the diagnosis of diabetes. The OGTT involves drinking a sugary beverage that contains 75 grams of glucose. The blood sugar is then tested several times in the next three hours to monitor the effects of the sugary drink on the blood sugar.

Complications

We've all heard horror stories about the complications that can occur from poorly controlled diabetes. I'm not discussing them here as a scare tactic. I don't think fear is a good motivator. Keep in mind that many people who have developed complications in the past may not have had access to proper treatment. After all, home blood sugar meters have only been available since the early 1980s, and blood sugar monitoring is an important tool in achieving control. There has been an explosion of new medications and treatment technologies for diabetes in the past couple of decades. Scientific studies have proven the benefits of proper diet and exercise in treating diabetes. We know more now about treating diabetes than ever before and are poised and ready to take control of this disease.

> Proper treatment can greatly reduce the risk of suffering ill effects from diabetes.

It's important to take diabetes seriously, because uncontrolled diabetes can lead to the following complications:

Diabetic ketoacidosis (DKA): DKA is a complication most commonly associated with type 1 diabetes. It occurs because of a lack of insulin. People with type 1 diabetes don't make any insulin. If they don't inject an appropriate amount of insulin, their bodies cannot use glucose properly. When the body is forced to burn fat during a relative shortage of insulin, ketones form as a by-product. Ketones are acidic and in large amounts can lead to coma or death.

Rarely, a person with type 2 diabetes can get diabetic ketoacidosis. When it does occur, it's usually in response to some other serious medical event such as a heart attack or severe infection, which has led to an imbalance of hormones in the body.

Hyperglycemic hyperosmolar nonketotic syndrome (HHNS):
With HHNS, blood sugar levels become extremely high (usually over
800 mg/dl), which changes the concentration of the blood. Symptoms
are thirst, frequent urination, dehydration, and lethargy, which leads
to confusion and changes in mental status. If left untreated, HHNS
can result in coma and death. It occurs more often in people with type
2 diabetes, particularly the elderly. Blood sugar monitoring can catch
and correct this problem in the early stages.

Hypoglycemia (low blood sugar): Low blood sugar may result from
some of the medications that are used to treat diabetes. See chapter 2
for a review of medications that may cause low blood sugar. See chapter 17 for complete guidelines on treating low blood sugar.

Eye damage: Complications to the eyes include diabetic retinopathy,
glaucoma, and cataracts. Retinopathy refers to damage of the retina,
which is the back of the eye. Retinopathy is essentially free of symptoms, which is why regular visits to the ophthalmologist (eye specialist)
are so important. Glaucoma is a change in the pressure in the eye.
Cataracts affect the lens of the eye.

Kidney damage: Damage to the kidney is known as nephropathy. A
simple urine test is used to diagnose kidney damage.

Nerve damage: Damage to the nerves is known as neuropathy. One
type of neuropathy is called distal polyneuropathy and it affects the
lower extremities—the feet and hands. It may result in burning, tin-
gling, or loss of sensation. Another type of neuropathy is autonomic
neuropathy, which is to blame for impotence, digestive disorders, problems with the bladder, and problems with the nerves that affect the
heart. Neuropathy can also impair sweating, which can cause dry,
cracked skin.

Infections: High blood sugar provides a nice sweet meal for bacteria,
yeast, and fungus to thrive on. High blood sugar also interferes with
the immune system's natural defenses for fighting infection.

Blood vessel disease: Poorly controlled diabetes increases your chance of heart disease, heart attack, stroke, or clogging of the blood vessels in your legs (peripheral vascular disease).

Periodontal disease: People with diabetes are more likely to have problems with infected gums and resultant tooth loss.

Foot problems: When several of the complications previously listed occur together, it can mean trouble for your feet. If you have decreased sensation in your feet because of neuropathy, you might injure your foot unknowingly. If your circulation is impaired because of blood vessel disease, then proper oxygen and nutrients are not as available to help heal the injury. Infections can occur because high blood sugar creates a perfect environment for bacteria to thrive, and your immune cells that are supposed to fight infection cannot work properly when your blood sugar is too high. Take good care of your feet! Be prompt in reporting any abnormalities to your doctor.

> High-fat diets and sedentary lifestyles have caused an alarming increase in childhood obesity, which has contributed to type 2 diabetes striking our young.

Remember, controlling your diabetes can drastically reduce your chances of complications. Learn about your diabetes. Take care of yourself. Choose to be well!

CHAPTER 2

Paths to Control

✐

IN THIS CHAPTER

- Introducing the diabetes team
- A healthful diet and exercise—the foundation to treating type 2 diabetes
- Diabetes medications
- Monitoring blood sugar
- The check-up checklist
- Personal health-care log

I f you want diabetes to treat you right, you have to treat your diabetes right. Diabetes is a chronic illness that requires ongoing attention. Controlling your blood sugar greatly reduces the chances of developing complications from diabetes. First, make sure you get the right information—then apply it!

People with diabetes benefit by receiving education and medical care from a team of health-care professionals that specializes in diabetes management. Your diabetes team can provide you with up-to-date information on diet, exercise, blood sugar monitoring, medications, and other medical therapies. The more you know, the more you can take charge of your own diabetes. After all, the most important person on your diabetes team is *you!*

Introducing the Diabetes Team

You are the central person on your diabetes team. The health-care professionals are your consultants. They can do much to assist you in your health care by providing information and setting up treatment plans, but the day-to-day care is your own responsibility. Ultimately, *you* must juggle diet, exercise, blood sugar monitoring, medications, and other self-care strategies. Enlist the support of family members and friends. The more support, the better!

Following is a list of potential health-care allies and a brief description of their role in your diabetes care.

- *The Primary Care Physician or Nurse Practitioner:* This team member oversees your total health care and may be responsible for referring you to other specialists. Sometimes primary care physicians or nurse practitioners medically manage your diabetes, and sometimes they refer you to a diabetes specialist.

- *The Endocrinologist:* An endocrinologist is a doctor who specializes in diseases of the endocrine system, including diabetes. If an endocrinologist is available to you, consult with this expert regarding your condition.

- *The Diabetes Nurse Educator:* This team member provides education on self–blood sugar monitoring and evaluating the results. The diabetes nurse educator teaches insulin administration, appropriate treatment of low blood sugar, travel tips, exercise issues, and handling of sick days. Other self-care strategies may be addressed as needed.

- *The Registered Dietitian:* This team member specializes in nutrition and diet therapies for diabetes and other health issues. The registered dietitian is the expert trained to individualize nutrition prescriptions to your needs and assist you with practical ways to implement those tips. Dietitians can also provide strategies for problems such as obesity, high blood pressure, and high cholesterol. Tips for treating low blood sugar and balancing diet and exercise are also topics they cover.

- *The Social Worker, Counselor, or Mental Health Specialist:* This person specializes in helping you to cope with a chronic illness. Stress and depression can interfere with your ability to perform ongoing self-care strategies and can ultimately sabotage your self-care. If you feel overwhelmed, excessively stressed, or think that you're depressed, ask your primary care physician or nurse practitioner for a referral to a mental health specialist.

- *The Podiatrist:* This doctor specializes in caring for your feet.

- *The Ophthalmologist:* This doctor specializes in examining and caring for your eyes.

- *The Pharmacist:* The pharmacist can answer your questions about prescription drugs and over-the-counter medications.

- *The Exercise Physiologist:* An exercise physiologist makes sure that your exercise routine is designed to safely meet your needs.

- *The Dentist and Dental Hygienist:* They provide care for your teeth and gums.

A Healthful Diet and Exercise— the Foundation to Treating Type 2 Diabetes

Proper diet and regular exercise are the foundation treatments for type 2 diabetes. Any other management strategies are built on top of this foundation. Taking medication for your diabetes doesn't mean that you can disregard your diet or exercise strategies. Each strategy is one piece of the puzzle, and all pieces of the puzzle fit together.

One way to stay on track with your diet and exercise plan is to periodically keep a food and activity log (see figure 2.1). Try

> Ultimately, *you* must juggle diet, exercise, blood sugar monitoring, medications, and other self-care strategies.

writing down everything that you eat and drink for a few days. Keep track of your exercise sessions. Review your records. Record keeping really helps you to pay attention to your day-to-day routine. Look for ways to improve your eating and exercise habits. Food and activity records should be shared with your diabetes team members. The more they know about your usual eating and activity patterns, the more useful they will be in helping to design treatment plans.

When you record your foods and beverages, it helps to write down the portion sizes. The sample food and activity log also encourages you to make comments that might be relevant to your meal or snack intake. You may choose to list the time of the meal, where it was eaten, if it was a special occasion meal or a restaurant meal, or even if you realized that you were eating out of boredom! You may use the comment section to track the grams of carbohydrate eaten, grams of fat, or calories.

Tip: Bring your records to your medical visits.

Figure 2.1—Food and Activity Log

Food and Activity	Date:
Breakfast:	Comments:
Snack:	Comments:
Lunch:	Comments:
Snack:	Comments:
Dinner:	Comments:
Snack:	Comments:
Exercise: (type and duration)	

Diabetes Medications

If proper diet and regular exercise fail to completely control the diabetes, medications should be added to help you control your blood sugar.

Requiring medication doesn't mean that you have failed at dietary management. Some individuals require medication regardless of how much effort they put into their diet and exercise plan.

There are several classes of medication, and each type works differently. Medications may be used alone or in combination to achieve the desired results. Sometimes

> Stress and depression can interfere with your ability to perform ongoing self-care strategies and can ultimately sabotage your self-care.

insulin is used for control of type 2 diabetes. The following summary will introduce you to some of the most common medications available today. Keep your eyes and ears open, as new medications are continually being developed and released.

Oral Agents: Diabetes Pills

This brief introduction describes the main medications available at this time. Your health-care provider can evaluate which medication is best for you, as well as answer your questions regarding safety and side effects. The following information lists some of the main side effects but is not meant to be all-inclusive. If you take a medication that can cause low blood sugar, be sure to review chapter 17 to learn more about preventing and treating low blood sugar.

Tip: If you forget to take your diabetes pill, don't double up on the next dose.

Sulfonylurea (sul-fa-nul-ur-ee-ah)

Examples: Glyburide (Micronase, Diabeta, Glynase), Glipizide (Glucotrol, Glucotrol XL), Glimepiride (Amaryl), Tolbutamide (Orinase), Tolazamide (Tolinase, Tolamide), Chlorpropamide (Diabinese), Acetohexamide (Dymelor)

How they work: Sulfonylureas work by stimulating your pancreas to produce more insulin. Some sulfonylureas also make the body's cells more sensitive to insulin.

Side effects: Risk for low blood sugar, so do not skip meals. Potential weight gain.

Meglitinide (meg-lit-in-ide)

Examples: Repaglinide (Prandin)

How they work: Meglitinides work by stimulating your pancreas to produce more insulin for the meal that is about to be eaten. The medication should be taken within 30 minutes before the meal.

Side effects: Risk for low blood sugar. Do not skip meals.

Phenylalanine Derivative (fe-nol-al-a-neen)

Examples: Nateglinide (Starlix)

How they work: When taken before a meal, phenylalanine derivatives stimulate rapid insulin production to control blood sugar peaks that occur after the meal.

Side effects: There is a small risk for low blood sugar.

Biguanide (bi-gwan-ide)

Examples: Metformin (Glucophage)

How they work: Biguanides decrease the amount of stored sugar that is released from the liver. They also help to improve insulin sensitivity so that the body responds to its own insulin better.

One way to stay on track with your diet and exercise plan is to periodically keep a food and activity log.

Side effects: Do not typically cause low blood sugar. Might cause nausea, loss of appetite, upset stomach, gas, or diarrhea, which may resolve in time. Lactic acidosis, a serious complication, occurs very rarely. You should not take this drug if you have kidney disease, liver disease, or congestive heart failure.

Thiazolidinedione (thigh-ah-zo-la-deen-dye-own)

Examples: Rosiglitazone (Avandia), Pioglitazone (Actos)

How they work: Thiazolidinediones decrease insulin resistance. They help the glucose get out of the bloodstream and into the individual cells where it is needed.

Side effects: Do not typically cause low blood sugar. Cannot be used if you have any type of liver disease. Might result in liver toxicity, so the drug requires frequent blood lab tests to monitor liver function. Might cause fluid retention or anemia.

Alpha-Glucosidase Inhibitor (alfa-glue-kos-a-dase)

Examples: Acarbose (Precose), Miglitol (Glyset)

How they work: Alpha-glucosidase inhibitors slow down the absorption of some types of carbohydrate in the intestine. Because the carbohydrate foods get absorbed more slowly, the blood sugar level after the meal doesn't go as high.

Side effects: The main complaints are intestinal gas, diarrhea, and cramping, which might resolve in time. This medication does *not* cause low blood sugar but, if you take it in addition to a sulfonylurea or a meglitinide—which *can* cause low blood sugar—then it is important to treat the low blood sugar with glucose tablets. Alpha-glucosidase inhibitors slow the absorption of sugar and starch, so those forms of carbohydrate would not sufficiently correct a low blood sugar reaction.

Insulin

Insulin is a hormone that is made by the pancreas. As the body's storage hormone, it has the important job of helping to use and store carbohydrate, protein, and fat. People with type 2 diabetes still make insulin, but sometimes they may need to take supplemental insulin injections to achieve better blood sugar control. As many as 40 percent of people with type 2 diabetes take insulin injections.

If you take insulin, it is important to be aware of *when* the insulin works. Table 2.1 lists the common types of human insulin preparations currently available. Review the timing schedules for any insulin that you use. The *start* time indicates how long it takes for the particular insulin to begin to work, the *peak* time illustrates when the insulin is working its hardest to lower your blood sugar, and the *duration* gives you an idea of how long the insulin works.

Tip: The insulin action times in table 2.1 are approximates. For some types of insulin, the size of the dose may affect the onset, peak, and duration times.

Table 2.1   Insulin Action

Type of Insulin	Start	Peak	Duration
Rapid Acting			
Humalog "Lispro"	5–15 minutes	30–90 minutes	2–4 hours
Novolog "Aspart"	5–15 minutes	30–90 minutes	2–4 hours
Short Acting			
Regular	30–60 minutes	2–3 hours	3–6 hours
Intermediate Acting			
NPH	2–4 hours	4–10 hours	10–16 hours
Lente	3–4 hours	4–12 hours	12–18 hours
Long Acting			
Ultralente	6–10 hours	no peak	18–20 hours
Glargine	1 hour	no peak	24 hours

Premixed Insulin

Many people with type 2 diabetes take premixed insulin, which consists of two kinds of insulin mixed into one vial. A short-acting insulin is mixed with an intermediate-acting insulin. The short-acting insulin may be regular insulin or lispro insulin, while the intermediate-acting insulin may be either NPH or NPL. (NPL is only available in premixed insulin preparations. It is not sold separately.)

- **70/30 insulin** is a mixture containing 70 percent NPH and 30 percent regular insulin. That means if you were to take 10 units of 70/30, you would actually be getting 7 units of NPH and 3 units of regular insulin.

- **50/50 insulin** is a mixture containing 50 percent NPH and 50 percent regular insulin. In this case, a dose of 10 units would end up being 5 units of NPH and 5 units of regular insulin.

- **75/25 insulin** is a mixture containing 75 percent NPL and 25 percent lispro insulin. Taking 10 units of this solution would provide you with 7½ units of NPL and 2½ units of lispro.

Timing is everything

When using premixed insulin, keep in mind that the short-acting insulin covers the meal about to be eaten. The long-acting insulin kicks in a bit later and works to cover the next meal. Insulin doses and meals have to be timed in order to maximize blood sugar control, as well as prevent low blood sugar. You should never skip meals when using insulin. To do so could cause significant hypoglycemia (low blood sugar).

> The fact that you checked your blood sugar is *good*, no matter what the results are.

- **70/30 and 50/50 insulin** should be taken about 30 minutes before the pending meal. The next meal should be eaten 4–5 hours later. For example, people who take 70/30 or 50/50 before breakfast should take the shot 30 minutes before they sit down to eat breakfast. Then lunch should be eaten 4–5 hours later.

- **75/25 insulin** can be taken just prior to eating. Once the injection has been taken, it is important to eat within 15 minutes. The following meal should be eaten 4–5 hours later.

When you take premixed insulin before dinner, you should not need to eat in the middle of the night. The intermediate-acting portion of the insulin is used to control the sugar that is released from your liver while you sleep.

Insulin Storage and Safety

Insulin can be stored at room temperature for up to 1–2 months. Keep extra, unopened bottles of insulin in the refrigerator, not the freezer. Because temperature extremes will inactivate insulin, you should avoid leaving it in direct sunlight or in a hot car. You should not use insulin that is past its expiration date. If your clear insulin (Humalog, Novolog, or Regular) becomes cloudy, it has become contaminated and should be thrown out. If your cloudy insulin (NPH, Lente, Ultralente, or Glargine) becomes clumpy, it should be discarded.

Final Comments Regarding the Use of Medications for Your Diabetes

No matter which type of medication or combination of medications you use, it is important that you take your pills or insulin in the manner prescribed by your health-care provider. Errors in the timing or the dose can increase your risk for side effects, so make sure that your health-care team has answered all of your medication questions.

Medication doses may need to be increased or decreased over time, depending on many variables. Be sure to see your health-care team regularly to review your regimen.

Monitoring your blood sugar at home will provide you with information on how well you are controlling your diabetes. Be sure to let your health-care provider know if you have blood sugar levels that are either too high or too low. Anytime you experience hypoglycemia (low blood sugar) it is important that you eat or drink some carbohydrates to quickly raise your blood sugar level. See chapter 17 for more information on treating low blood sugar.

Monitoring Blood Sugar

Blood sugar monitoring provides information about how your diabetes is doing. Don't think of the numbers as "good" or "bad." The fact that you checked your blood sugar is *good*, no matter what the results are. If the number is above target, you can choose to do something about it. I can't tell you how many people have come to their clinic appointments and have made up numbers to write in their logbooks. They didn't want to write the high numbers down, so they made up numbers that

> Home blood sugar monitoring is extremely important. Urine testing for glucose is obsolete.

they thought were better. Kids do it because they want to please their parents. Adolescents do it because sometimes they forget to test or don't want to test as often as they are told to. I've even seen parents make up numbers in their child's logbook because they were afraid the medical team would judge them for not being able to better control their child's diabetes. I've seen pregnant women make up numbers to fool the team because they didn't want to go on insulin. Some adults have done it because they didn't know how to work the monitor and were too embarrassed to ask for help. Whatever the reason, don't do it! There is no shame in having diabetes. Truthful, accurate blood sugar logs are *critical* in making decisions regarding treatment. The goal is to take good care of the diabetes. If the team members don't know what the blood sugar is doing, they can't be aggressive in managing the diabetes.

Your blood sugar should be monitored when you go to your clinic visits, but it is also extremely important that you monitor your levels in your own home. Urine testing for glucose is obsolete; it does not give an accurate representation of the current blood sugar levels because urine accumulates in the bladder over time. Testing the urine tells if sugar went into the urine in the previous hours but doesn't let you know how much sugar is in the blood at any specific moment. Only blood sugar monitoring can tell you that.

Most people with diabetes are advised to try to keep their blood sugar levels as close to normal as possible. Be sure to ask your health-care provider for guidelines on what *your* target blood sugar range should be. Your health-care provider should consider your age, your medications, and your other medical conditions when setting treatment goals and blood sugar targets. The following is provided for reference only. Numbers are listed in milligrams per deciliter. (If you are more familiar with millimoles per liter, you can convert mg/d to mmol/l by dividing by 18.) These values reflect plasma-referenced meters (most meters are plasma referenced). If you use a meter that reports its values as whole blood, then your targets would be approximately 10 percent lower. If you aren't certain which type of meter that you have, you can call the toll-free number on the back of the meter to find out. Note: These values pertain to *nonpregnant* adults.

> Your blood sugar level changes throughout the day in relation to your meals, medications, and activity. Stress, pain, and illness can also cause your blood sugar to fluctuate.

Blood Sugar Values (mg/dl)

Before Meals

Normal is less than 110.

Goal is usually 90–130.

Corrective action is usually recommended if the number is less than 90 or over 150.

1–2 Hours After Meals

Normal is less than 140.

Goal varies according to your medications and your medical history, but the closer to normal, the better. Your provider can help you set your target. Some providers set the upper limit target at 180, while others strive for 160. If your blood sugar after meals frequently exceeds 200, then you should speak to your health-care provider about treatment options.

Bedtime

Normal is less than 120.

Goal is usually 110–150.

Corrective action is usually recommended if the number is less than 110 or over 180.

If your numbers frequently fall into the *corrective action* range, you should seek medical advice. You may need therapy adjustments.

Home Blood Sugar Monitoring

Why Should You Self-Monitor Your Blood Sugar?

Because if you don't know what your blood sugar level is, then you don't know how well your diabetes is being controlled. And what you don't know *can* hurt you. Your blood sugar level changes throughout the day in relation to your meals, medications, and activity (see figure 2.2). Stress, pain, and illness can also cause your blood sugar to fluctuate. Checking your blood sugar at various times of the day can give you a snapshot view of what's happening with your blood sugar at that exact moment.

Figure 2.2—Blood Sugar Profile Curves

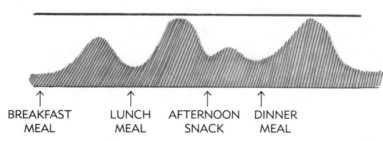

BREAKFAST   LUNCH   AFTERNOON   DINNER
MEAL   MEAL   SNACK   MEAL

Figure 2.3—Blood Sugar Meters

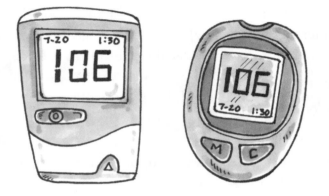

Only a very small drop of blood is required. It is obtained with a tiny lancing device. Most lancing devices are used to prick the fingers (you should start by washing your hands with warm soapy water!), though some allow blood to be obtained from other areas of the body (such as the forearm) where there are less nerve endings. The drop of blood is applied to a test strip, which is inserted into the meter. The meter reads the blood sugar level and provides results in less than a minute.

Choosing a Meter

People with diabetes should have their own blood sugar meters. It's important to be properly trained on the use of the meter. If you don't have a meter, ask your doctor for one and for instruction on its use. A diabetes educator can show you various meters and help you to decide which meter is the best for your needs.

Insurance companies are sometimes picky about which meter and supplies they will pay for, so be sure to get a meter that your health plan accepts.

Many meters are on the market. They are all pretty small and easy to use, some easier than others. Most meters have a memory and retain a record of your blood sugar results. Some meters allow you to download the data to a computer, which will give you printouts and graphs to help you and your doctor evaluate the results. Other meters have data management systems that allow you to record events such as meal carbohydrate grams eaten, exercise, or insulin doses received. Meters are available for the visually impaired. A clear, step-by-step voice prompts the visually impaired person through the testing procedure. The technology is impressive. You may want a simple meter that gives you step-by-step cues on performing the test, or you may want a meter with all the bells and whistles. But either way, get a meter!

Meters operate within a reasonable margin of error. If you did two blood sugar tests right in a row, it's unlikely that you would get the exact same results. The numbers could be within 5 to 10 percent of each other, and that would still be considered within the meter's range of accuracy. Meters usually come with a special check strip that you can insert into the meter to make sure

> Insurance companies are sometimes picky about which meter and supplies they will pay for, so be sure to get a meter that your health plan accepts.

it is working properly. Control solutions are available to use with your test strips to check meter performance. The control solution is used in place of blood to check the accuracy of the meter. Most meters require you to program a "code" into the meter to match the current batch of test strips that you are using. Every time you get another supply of strips, you need to change the code. Failing to do so can interfere with your meter's ability to provide accurate results. Another thing to keep in mind is that your test strips need to be kept in the vial or package they came in until you're ready to use them. If you take strips out of the package, they are exposed to light and moisture, which can ruin them, and they might not provide accurate test results.

Tip: You should periodically check the accuracy of your meter by running a control solution check. Refer to your meter's instruction manual, ask your health-care provider for help, or call the toll-free number on the back of your meter.

Whole Blood Versus Plasma

When you test your blood at home, you use whole blood. When you get a blood test at the lab, technicians use plasma, which is the fluid from the blood after the blood cells are removed. Home blood glucose meters come calibrated to either whole blood or plasma. What that means is that plasma-referenced meters will provide results consistent with the results you'd get if you had your blood drawn at a lab. By comparison, whole blood readings are about 10–15 percent lower than plasma readings.

When Should You Test?

Your health-care provider can help you decide when and how often to check your blood sugar. You may be asked to check anywhere from one to four times per day. Some individuals who are well controlled without the use of medications may only need to check their blood sugar several times per week. It's a good idea to vary the times of the day that you check your sugar, in order to get a more complete picture of what happens throughout the day. Common times to check blood sugar levels are as follows:

- *Fasting blood sugar.* This blood sugar check is done first thing in the morning before you eat anything. (For a true fasting value, you should not have eaten anything for at least 8 hours.) Fasting blood sugar checks let you know how well your blood sugar has been controlled overnight while you sleep. They also let you know if your hormones are driving your blood sugar levels up. Hormones cause the liver to release stored sugar. The "dawn phenomenon" refers to the hormonally driven elevated blood sugar levels that occur in the early morning hours.

- *Before and after meal* blood sugar checks let you know how you respond to the foods that you eat. Any time you want to see how you respond to a particular meal or food, you can check your blood sugar before you eat it, and then check it again about an hour after eating. It can be enlightening!

- *Occasionally*, *check at 2:00 or 3:00 A.M.*, if you are taking insulin or pills that work overnight. This check can ensure that your dose of medication is adequate, yet not so strong that it's causing low blood sugar while you sleep.

- *Before and after exercise* blood sugar checks let you know how your body responds to physical activity. You'll find it very rewarding to see how exercise can improve your blood sugar levels. You might also be alerted to blood sugar levels that drop too low from the combination of exercise and medications.

- *Before you drive a car.* If you take medications that can cause low blood sugar, checking your blood sugar before you get behind the wheel is an important safety measure.

- *Symptoms of low blood sugar.* Check your blood sugar any time you suspect that it is too low.

- *During illness.* Check your blood sugar more often if you are sick. Illness can cause blood sugar to go up.

Record Your Blood Sugar Results

Use a logbook to record your blood sugar values (see figure 2.4). Your health-care provider doesn't want to scroll through your meter's memory, number by number, to review your results. A logbook offers the added

> If you have poor sensation in your feet, then you have to be especially careful to avoid injury.

benefit of organizing your blood sugar readings into the various times of the day that you check. It allows both you and your health-care team to see patterns in your blood sugar levels. In other words, you might have certain times of the day when your blood sugar is not well controlled. When a reproducible pattern is observed, a treatment plan can be instituted. Once you, yourself, notice a pattern that indicates inadequate

Figure 2.4—Blood Sugar Log Form

Day	Date	Breakfast		Lunch		Dinner		Bed	Other	Comments
		pre	post	pre	post	pre	post			
Sun										
Mon										
Tue										
Wed										
Thu										
Fri										
Sat										
Sun										
Mon										
Tue										
Wed										
Thu										
Fri										
Sat										

control, then call your health-care provider to get advice on ways to improve your control. Medication doses may need to be adjusted. Be proactive. Don't wait months for your next appointment if you notice that your diabetes isn't being controlled. The sooner you seek help, the sooner you can regain control of your diabetes.

Lab Tests That Measure Long-Term Control of Blood Sugar

Hemoglobin A1c

What it is. Hemoglobin A1c (HbA1c) is a blood test that can give you an estimate of your *average* blood sugar control over the past 2–3 months. It's like taking a motion picture of all the blood sugar variations, the highs, and the lows, and giving you the *average* for the past 2- to 3-month period. (Using your home blood glucose monitor is still important to get the "snapshot" view of specific blood sugar values.)

How often to get it done. It's recommended that people with type 2 diabetes have this test done every 3 months until their diabetes is controlled and stable. Then the HbA1c test should be repeated at least every 6 months. Write yourself a reminder on your calendar. It's unlikely that anyone else will come knocking on your door to make sure that the test gets done!

How it works. The HbA1c test analyzes the amount of glucose that has permanently attached to your red blood cells. When blood glucose levels go up too high and stay up, then more glucose gets attached to the blood cells. Since red blood cells last about 120 days, this test shows a picture of blood sugar control over the life of the blood cell. Not all blood cells are replaced in the body at the same time. So, at any given time, you have some blood cells that are new, some that are a month old, some that are two months old, and so on. The HbA1c is most representative of the blood sugar control over the past 2–3 months.

> Controlling your blood sugar greatly reduces the chances of developing complications from diabetes.

What the results mean. HbA1c test results are expressed in percentages. What is considered "normal" varies from lab to lab, depending on its test procedure. *Compare your test results to your lab's normal ranges.*

Someone who does not have diabetes would have a HbA1c value somewhere between 4 and 6 percent. The American Diabetes Association recommends that people with diabetes achieve a value less than 7 percent. Any value above 8 percent warrants a reevaluation of treatment and *action.*

Table 2.2 shows you the *average* blood sugar level that corresponds to the HbA1c results. *This chart holds true if your lab's normal range is 4–6 percent.*

Table 2.2 What's Your Average?

HbA1c	Corresponding Average Blood Sugar (mg/dl)
4	60
5	90
6	120
7	150
8	180
9	210
10	240
11	270
12	300
13	330
14	360

Fructosamine Test

The fructosamine test analyzes a different substance in the blood but works pretty much the same way as the HbA1c test. However, it gives a picture of the average blood sugar control over the past 2–3 *weeks*, whereas the HbA1c gives a picture of the past 2–3 months.

The Check-Up Checklist

The Physical Exam

You should get a complete physical exam every year. Your doctor may choose to do certain tests more frequently than that. Some issues that should be addressed at your annual check-up include:

- Diabetes management, including blood sugar control and medications

- Lipid levels, such as total cholesterol, LDL cholesterol, HDL cholesterol, triglycerides

- Blood pressure

- Weight

- Flu shot

- Additional blood work, labs, or tests, as determined by the health-care provider

- Additional questions or concerns that you have

Diabetes Follow-Up Visits

Besides your annual physical exam, your diabetes management must be followed regularly. The frequency of your medical visits depends upon your blood sugar control, medications, and risk or presence of complications. Quarterly visits are usually recommended until treatment goals are achieved. If your diabetes is poorly controlled, you may need to be seen more

> It's recommended that people with type 2 diabetes have a hemoglobin A1c test done every 3 months until their diabetes is controlled and stable, and every 6 months thereafter.

frequently. Be sure to bring your blood sugar records and your blood sugar meter to your check-ups. You can also bring any food records or exercise logs that you have kept. Blood pressure and weight should be monitored at every visit.

The Feet

Put your right foot forward and take strides in preventing foot problems. Your feet work hard for you, carrying you around day after day. Don't forget to give them a little tender loving care. Uncontrolled diabetes can lead to circulatory problems and nerve damage, which can leave your feet vulnerable to injury.

Figure 2.5—Foot Exam

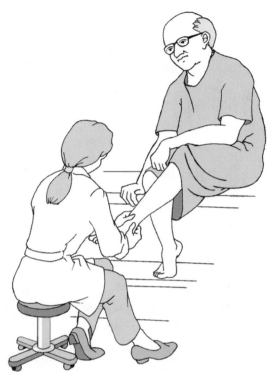

Foot Exams

- Look at your own feet every day. Report blisters, sores, injuries, discolored skin, or any other abnormal situations to your doctor right away.

- Have your doctor look at your feet at every office visit.

- Have your doctor perform a complete foot exam at least once a year.

Wear Comfortable, Well-Fitting Socks and Shoes

Socks should fit comfortably . . . not too big, not too small. Choose seamless socks or socks with seams that lie flat and don't form lumps. For exercise, choose soft, padded socks that wick moisture away from your feet.

Shoes should be comfortable at the time you buy them. You shouldn't have to "break them in." Let an experienced shoe salesperson assist you in finding a proper fit. A podiatrist can assess your need for arch supports, orthotics, or therapeutic shoes.

If you have poor sensation in your feet, then you have to be especially careful to avoid injury. Don't go barefoot. Wear something protective on your feet, such as slippers, even in the house. Don't use heating pads on your feet. Test bath water temperature with your elbow before putting your feet in the tub. See a podiatrist for additional foot-care guidelines.

The Eyes

You should have a complete eye exam by an ophthalmologist every year. The pupils must be dilated to view the back of the eye (the retina). This painless test should be performed when you are first diagnosed with type 2 diabetes, and then again every year afterward. Treatments are available if eye damage is detected early. Don't put this off!

The Kidneys

A simple urine test can detect early stages of kidney damage. Testing for microalbumin (which means small amounts of protein in the urine) can let you and your doctor know how your kidneys are doing. This test should be performed when you are first diagnosed with type 2 diabetes, and then again every year afterward. Be sure to ask your doctor for this test.

Figure 2.6—The Eye

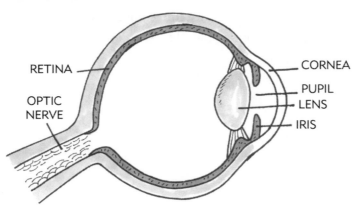

Figure 2.7—The Kidneys

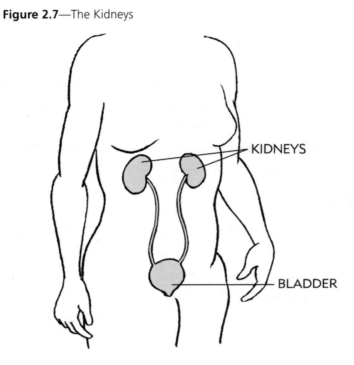

KIDNEYS

BLADDER

Your health-care provider may also do blood tests that assess kidney health. BUN (blood urea nitrogen), serum creatinine, and creatinine clearance are tests used to track the health of the kidneys.

Dental Care

Diabetes may increase your risk for gum infections. Brushing twice a day and flossing once a day can reduce your chances of having problems with your teeth and gums. Have a dental check-up and teeth cleaning twice a year.

Figure 2.8—Personal Health-Care Log

Personal Health-Care Log					
Remember to bring meter, blood sugar logbook, and food records to clinic visits					
Clinic Visit Date:					
Complete Physical Exam					
Reviewed Blood Sugar Logbook					
Reviewed Medications					
Weight					
Blood Pressure (should be below 130/80)					
Hemoglobin A1c (should be below 7)					
Microalbumin (should be below 30)					
Total Cholesterol (should be below 200)					
LDL Cholesterol (should be below 100)					
HDL Cholesterol (should be above 40)					
Triglycerides (should be below 150)					
Other Important Labs:					
Other Important Labs:					
Prescriptions Renewed					
Flu Shot					
Complete Foot Exam					
Dilated Eye Exam					
Dental Exam and Teeth Cleaning					
Session with Nurse Educator					
Session with Registered Dietitian					
Session with Mental Health Specialist					
Other appointments:					
I have had an exercise stress test:	Yes/No				
I have medical alert identification:	Yes/No				

CHAPTER 3

Basic Nutrition Principles

❧

IN THIS CHAPTER

- The goals of Medical Nutrition Therapy for people with diabetes
- Dietary guidelines
- Fiber
- Importance of water
- Highlights on nutrition guidelines for Americans

S ome individuals who come to see me about their diets do so because *their doctor insisted.* They walk into my office with their arms folded across their chests and "I don't want to be here" written across their foreheads. Others have had negative past experiences with previous dietitians or health-care providers or have received little or no information regarding nutrition principles. How about you? Have you ever received a tear-off diet instruction sheet and no support to go with it? Or worse yet, have you tried to wade through the piles of diet books on the market? One book says to eat plenty of carbohydrates. Another book says to strictly limit carbohydrates. There is so much conflicting information! Have you noticed how people you know think they are experts in the field of nutrition and don't hesitate to advise what you should and shouldn't eat? It's no wonder that so many people with diabetes are confused and frustrated about what to eat. It shouldn't be that complicated. And, in fact, it isn't. It all boils down to eating healthful foods in appropriate amounts. Start with healthful eating habits, learn a few tools to tailor your diet to your diabetes, and you might find that things aren't as bad as you thought they'd be. Instead of focusing on *what you can't eat*, you may be pleased to find out *what you can eat*.

The word *diet* has negative connotations for many people. It implies that you'll have to give something up. I like to think of the word as something more holistic. Our diet is what we nourish ourselves with. In many ways, we are what we eat. Food is our fuel. We build our bodily tissues from the nutrients that we take in. There is *no one perfect diet* that will work for every person with diabetes, so diet prescriptions must be tailored to the individual.

Recently, the phrase *Medical Nutrition Therapy* has been coined to describe the diet that best supports health and healing. Science has shown that proper nutrition is crucial in treating diabetes. Medical Nutrition Therapy for diabetes is best obtained from a registered dietitian. Ideally, people with diabetes should meet with a registered dietitian who can help them find a sensible approach to eating. (If available, choose a registered dietitian who is also a certified diabetes educator.)

The goals of Medical Nutrition Therapy for people with diabetes:

- To achieve and maintain appropriate blood glucose levels
- To achieve and maintain optimal lipid (cholesterol and blood fat) levels
- To achieve and maintain a reasonable body weight
- To provide appropriate calories to children for growth and development
- To provide appropriate calories for pregnancy and lactation
- To prevent, delay, and treat the complications that can occur with diabetes
- To improve overall health through optimal nutrition

Registered dietitians (RDs)

Registered dietitians (RDs) are health-care experts who have been trained specifically in nutrition therapy for health and disease. The RD has completed a stringent course of study, holds a college degree in nutritional science, has completed an internship, and has passed a national examination in order to receive those credentials. To find a dietitian in your area, call 1-800-366-1655.

Armed with the proper knowledge and support, you can implement the tools that are necessary to achieve these goals. The following recommendations are an overview. See the individual chapters on protein, carbohydrate, and fat to learn more about specific portions and calculations on how many grams of each you need.

Dietary Guidelines

Food can be broken down into three main categories: protein, fat, and carbohydrate. The first step is finding out how much you need from each category.

Certified diabetes educators (CDEs)

Certified diabetes educators (CDEs) are health-care providers who have a minimum of 2 years of practice in their field and a minimum of 1,000 hours of experience in diabetes patient education. They have taken and passed a national certification examination. Registered dietitians, registered nurses, occupational therapists, pharmacists, physical therapists, physicians, podiatrists, social workers, and physician assistants can all become certified diabetes educators.

Protein

Opinions vary regarding protein intake, according to which book you pick up at the bookstore, but I agree with the recommendations made by the American Diabetes Association (ADA). It currently recommends that somewhere between 10 and 20 percent of your calories should come from protein. Incidentally, that's similar to the amount of protein recommended for healthy adults, as established by the Food and Nutrition Board's recommended dietary allowances (RDAs). In other words, people with diabetes have similar protein requirements to the rest of the population. There are some reasons to restrict protein intake. Protein restriction for kidney disease is addressed in the chapter devoted in depth to protein, chapter 7.

> The word *diet* has negative connotations for many people. It implies that you will have to give something up.

Once 10–20 percent of your calories are allocated to protein, that leaves 80–90 percent to be distributed between fat and carbohydrate. The ADA doesn't give hard guidelines on just how much should go to fat versus carbohydrate. It recommends looking at each individual's circumstances when setting goals. Considerations should include weight, cholesterol profile, blood sugar control, and current eating habits.

Fat

For most people I recommend setting fat intake at, or below, 30 percent of total calories. (The range is usually 25–35 percent, based on other health considerations.) Many health agencies have set that same fat limit to help reduce the risk of disease, particularly heart disease. (See highlights on Nutrition Guidelines for Americans at the end of this chapter.) The type of fat consumed is also of importance. Monounsaturated fat (olive oil, canola oil, avocados, olives, and peanuts) should be the type chosen most often, and it can supply up to 20 percent of the total calories. Less than 7 percent of your calories should come from the artery-clogging saturated fats (animal fats and solid fats). Polyunsaturated fats (most vegetable oils) can provide up to 10 percent of your total calories. For more information and practical guidelines, see chapter 8, which is devoted to fat, and chapter 11, which focuses on heart health.

Carbohydrate

With 10–20 percent of the calories coming from protein and approximately 30 percent coming from fat, that leaves about 50–60 percent of the calories to be consumed from carbohydrates. Carbohydrate is what turns into sugar in the blood. This sugar, also known as blood glucose, is the body's main fuel source. We *need* to eat carbohydrates. It's important to eat the right amount at the right time. Carbohydrate has to be planned to balance exercise and activity, and it has to be coordinated with insulin and oral diabetes medications. Although different sources of carbohydrate may produce different blood sugar responses, the *amount* and *timing* of the carbohydrate eaten have the most influence on blood sugar levels. To learn more about managing carbohydrate intake, turn to chapter 6. Guidelines on sugar can be found in chapter 16.

Exceptions to the Rule

Some individuals need lower-fat diets. Lower-fat diets may be prescribed, along with overall caloric restriction and exercise, to promote weight loss. Lower-fat diets may also be prescribed to improve heart health. For example, fat may be limited to 25 percent of the daily calories, or less.

Table 3.1   Suggested Breakdown of Calories

Carbohydrate	50–60 percent
Protein	10–20 percent
Fat	approximately 30 percent

With protein 10–20 percent, the carbohydrate allowance may be a higher percentage, perhaps as much as 55–65 percent of the total calories. Higher carbohydrate intake is usually better tolerated if the carbohydrates come from high-fiber sources such as whole grains and legumes.

On the other hand, some individuals require a somewhat lower-carbohydrate/higher-fat intake, based on other health concerns. This type of diet plan is sometimes used for individuals with low HDL cholesterol levels (the good kind of cholesterol), or people who have *moderately* elevated triglycerides (blood fats) or elevated VLDL (very low-density lipoprotein, another undesirable blood fat). For example, approximately 45–50 percent of the calories could come from carbohydrate, 15–20 percent from protein, and the remaining 35 percent would come from fat. For people who follow this higher fat intake, it's important to focus on using the heart-healthier monounsaturated fats. The best sources of monounsaturated fat are olive oil, canola oil, olives, avocados, peanuts, and peanut oil.

> Recently, the phrase *Medical Nutrition Therapy* has been coined to describe the diet that best supports health and healing.

Pregnancy is another time that a woman with diabetes may benefit from a somewhat lower carbohydrate intake because tight blood sugar control is imperative for a healthy pregnancy outcome. See chapter 14 for tips on nutrition during pregnancy.

Fiber

Fiber is the part of the plant food that cannot be digested. A healthful intake of fiber may prevent certain diseases of the intestines and colon, including colon cancer. Fiber recommendations for people with diabetes are the same as for the general public, 20–35 grams per day from a variety of foods. Most Americans fall short of that recommended intake. Whole grains, fruits, and vegetables are all good sources of fiber. (See chapter 18 for more fiber facts.)

Importance of Water

Don't underestimate the importance of water. It often goes unmentioned, but water is essential to health. Water makes up about 50 percent of a woman's body weight and about 60 percent of a man's weight. Water lubricates and cushions. It transports nutrients throughout the body. It also carries waste products out of the body. Water is needed to regulate body temperature. Perspiration and evaporation cool an overheated system. We couldn't exist without regular replenishments of water.

Drink up! Drink at least eight glasses of water per day. Broth, herb tea, milk, and caffeine-free, non-alcoholic beverages can count toward your fluid intake.

Sometimes it may be necessary to drink even more than eight glasses per day. Fluid requirements increase in hot weather due to water lost to perspiration. Uncontrolled blood sugar also increases fluid requirements, since high blood sugar causes more frequent urination. Exercise increases fluid needs, as do illness and fever. Don't wait until you feel thirsty to drink. Some people, particularly the elderly, have a diminished sensation of thirst.

> Although different sources of carbohydrate may produce different blood sugar responses, the *amount* and *timing* of the carbohydrate eaten have the most influence on blood sugar levels.

Having Said That, What's Next?

Knowing what percentage of your calories to eat from each main food group is one thing, but how exactly do you implement that information? You need something more tangible than percentages. There are several different menu-planning tools. Some people will do fine with simple dietary guidelines, coupled with good common sense. Others benefit by learning more detailed portioning tools. Find out what works best for you. It will depend on your blood sugar control, weight history, and other health concerns you have. Carbohydrate counting and use of the exchange system are addressed in chapter 6. Protein portioning and recommendations are found in chapter 7. Fat gram information and tips can be found in chapter 8. Brush up on your label reading with the chapter devoted to understanding food labels, chapter 5.

Highlights on Nutrition Guidelines for Americans

The *Dietary Guidelines for Americans* established by the Department of Health and Human Services, in conjunction with the U.S. Department of Agriculture, recommend that no more than 30 percent of your calories should come from fat, and of that, no more than 10 percent should be saturated fat. They promote three or more servings of vegetables, two or more servings of fruit, and six or more servings from grains each day. They recommend minimizing sugar, salt, and alcohol use.

> A healthful intake of fiber may prevent certain diseases of the intestines and colon, including colon cancer.

The Report on Nutrition and Health by the Surgeon General basically agrees with the Dietary Guidelines for Americans. It also promotes weight control and exercise.

Healthy People 2000 from the U.S. Public Health Service also recommends that less than 30 percent of calories come from fat. It promotes 5 or more servings per day from a combination of fruits and vegetables, and 6 or more servings per day from grains, along with a decrease in salt intake.

The Food Guide Pyramid from the U.S. Department of Agriculture and the U.S. Department of Health and Human Services is a tool to help with meal planning. It recommends eating the following:

6–11 servings from the Bread, Cereal, Rice, and Pasta Group

3–5 servings from the Vegetable Group

2–4 servings from the Fruit Group

2–3 servings from the Milk and Yogurt Group

2–3 servings from the Meat, Poultry, Fish, Eggs, and Nuts Group

Use fats, oils, and sweets sparingly.

(Notice that the serving goals are given as a range. Your actual requirements depend upon your weight goals and your calorie needs.)

The National Cholesterol Education Program made the following diet recommendations a part of its Therapeutic Lifestyle Changes (TLC) diet for people with elevated cholesterol levels:

Fat should be 25–35 percent of total calories, composed of saturated fat less than 7 percent, polyunsaturated fat up to 10 percent, and monounsaturated fat up to 20 percent. Keep dietary cholesterol intake below 200 mg/day. Eat 50–60 percent of your calories as carbohydrate and approximately 15 percent of your calories from protein. Strive for 20–30 grams of fiber per day.

Personal Profile

༄

You don't have to count calories to watch what you eat. But having a rough idea of how many calories your body needs per day is useful information. That way, when you look at a food label and read the calories, you will at least have a reference point to help you choose wisely. Once you know your caloric needs, it's easy to determine how many grams of carbohydrate, protein, and fat you need each day. This chapter is designed to help you assess your caloric needs, as well as ideals in body weight.

Your Personal Assessment Data Form

As you read this chapter, you will be guided to calculate an appropriate weight for your height. Then, you can use the following assessment parameters to help determine your risk for obesity-related diseases: body mass index (BMI), waist circumference, and waist-hip ratio. Finally, you will be able to calculate an estimated number of calories to eat for *weight maintenance*. To adjust your calories for weight loss, first complete this chapter, and then see chapter 9, "Weight Matters."

Use the following form to record your values as you work through the chapter.

Personal Assessment Data Form

Weight for Height Calculation: _____
Body Mass Index (BMI): _____
BMI Category: _____
Waist Circumference: _____
Waist-Hip Ratio: _____
Calorie Level to Maintain Current Weight: _____

Calculating Appropriate Weight for Height

You've probably seen charts that tell you how much you should weigh for your height. Values vary somewhat between the charts. Calculations can also be done to get a general idea of an appropriate weight for your height. Charts and calculations are only ways to *estimate* reasonable weights. Keep in mind that most of these tools don't make adjustments for age or fitness level.

Use the following formula to calculate ideal body weight for height. *Don't let the results discourage you.* Individual variation exists and you may be perfectly healthy at an alternate weight. However, if your current weight exceeds the calculated weight by too much, then you could very well be at increased risk for obesity-related illnesses.

Women

Give yourself 100 pounds for the first 5 feet in height. Then, add 5 pounds for every additional inch over 5 feet. If you have a small frame, subtract 10 percent from that total. If you have a large frame, add 10 percent to that total.

Men

Give yourself 106 pounds for the first 5 feet in height. Then, add 6 pounds for every additional inch over 5 feet. If you have a small frame, subtract 10 percent from that total. If you have a large frame, add 10 percent to that total.

Body Mass Index (BMI)

Body mass index (BMI) uses weight and height to categorize level of body fat and risk profile for developing obesity-related diseases. To use the BMI table provided (table 4.1), find your height (in inches) along the left column. Then follow a straight line from your height until you find the weight that is closest to your own. Once you locate your weight, follow a straight line up to the top of the chart to find the number that corresponds to your BMI. The same table is used for both women and men.

Charts and calculations are only ways to *estimate* reasonable weights. Keep in mind that most of these tools don't make adjustments for age or fitness level.

The higher the BMI number is, the greater the risk of developing health problems related to obesity (see table 4.2). On the other hand, a BMI that is below normal can indicate health risks due to nutritional deficiencies.

Tip: For those of you who are more familiar with the metric system, you can convert as follows: 1 kilogram is equal to 2.2 pounds, and there are 2.54 centimeters to an inch.

Table 4.1   Body Mass Index Table

BMI	19	20	21	22	23	24	25	26	27	28	29	30	35	40
Height (inches)	**Weight (pounds)**													
58	91	96	100	105	110	115	119	124	129	134	139	143	167	191
59	94	99	104	109	114	119	124	129	133	138	143	148	173	198
60	97	102	107	112	118	123	128	133	138	143	148	153	179	204
61	100	106	111	116	122	127	132	137	143	148	153	158	185	211
62	104	109	115	120	126	131	136	142	147	153	158	164	191	218
63	107	113	118	124	130	135	141	147	152	158	163	169	197	225
64	111	116	122	128	134	140	145	151	157	163	169	174	204	233
65	114	120	126	132	138	144	150	156	162	168	174	180	210	240
66	118	124	130	136	142	148	155	161	167	173	179	186	216	247
67	121	127	134	140	147	153	159	166	172	178	185	191	223	255
68	125	131	138	144	151	158	164	171	177	184	190	197	230	263
69	128	135	142	149	155	162	169	176	183	189	196	203	237	270
70	132	139	146	153	160	167	174	181	188	195	202	209	243	278
71	136	143	150	157	165	172	179	186	193	200	208	215	250	286
72	140	147	155	162	169	177	184	191	199	206	213	221	258	294
73	144	151	159	166	174	182	189	197	204	212	219	227	265	303
74	148	155	163	171	179	187	194	202	210	218	225	233	272	311
75	152	160	168	176	184	192	200	208	216	224	232	240	279	319
76	156	164	172	180	189	197	205	213	221	230	238	246	287	328

* Body mass index is calculated as (kilograms of weight) divided by (height in meters)[2]

Table 4.2   BMI Categories

BMI below 18.5 is considered underweight.
BMI 18.5–24.9 is considered normal weight.
BMI 25.0–29.9 is considered overweight (increased risk).
BMI 30.0–34.9 is considered Grade 1 obesity (high risk).
BMI 35.0–39.9 is considered Grade 2 obesity (very high risk).
BMI 40 and above is considered Grade 3 obesity (extremely high risk).

Examples

- Pat is 5'7" (67 inches) and weighs 140 pounds. Pat has a BMI of 22, which is consistent with a normal weight for that height.

- Taylor is 5'8" (68 inches) and weighs 197 pounds. Taylor has a BMI of 30, which is considered Grade 1 obesity.

Limitations of BMI

BMI does not give an accurate representation of body composition when a person has an unusually large amount of muscle. For example, a body builder or a professional athlete might have a BMI consistent with obesity when, in fact, that person is actually heavier than average because of muscle weight. (Muscle, a healthy tissue, is denser than fat; therefore, muscle weighs more than fat.) On the other hand, BMI can underestimate body fat stores in a person who has lost lean muscle mass, such as an elderly individual. Finally, BMI does not always accurately assess body fat stores in individuals who are under 5 feet tall.

Body Fat Distribution and Health Risks

Being overweight can have many negative health consequences. *Where* you carry that extra weight matters. Body fat distribution determines

Figure 4.1—Apple and Pear Body Shapes

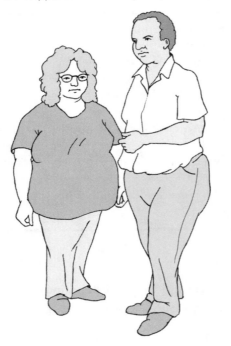

your risk profile for obesity-related diseases. Individuals who carry the extra pounds around their waists are described as "apple shaped," while those who carry the extra pounds around their hips are called "pear shaped" (see figure 4.1). The apple-shaped physique is associated with the highest risk for developing diabetes, heart disease, high blood pressure, and high blood lipids (cholesterol and blood fats).

To assess your own risk, you can measure your waist circumference or your waist-hip ratio.

Waist Circumference

To locate the correct position to place the measuring tape, act as if you were standing with your hands on your hips and feel for the top crest of the hip bones. Position the tape measure just above those bones and circle your waist with the tape measure parallel to the ground. Relax your stomach and breath normally. Keep the tape measure snug, but don't cause the skin to compress.

High Risk for Obesity-Related Diseases

Men: Waist circumference greater than 40 inches (102 cm)

Women: Waist circumference greater than 35 inches (88 cm)

Waist-Hip Ratio

With a tape measure, measure your waist as described previously in the section on waist circumference. Then measure your hips at the largest point. Waist measurement divided by hip measurement is the number you're looking for. When the number is greater than 1 in men and greater than 0.8 in women, the risk for disease increases.

> The apple-shaped physique is associated with the highest risk for developing diabetes, heart disease, and high blood pressure.

Example

Liz has a waist measurement of 42 inches. Her hip measurement is 39 inches. Waist measurement divided by hip measurement is 42 ÷ 39 = 1.08 (rounded to the nearest hundredth). Since this number is greater than 0.8 for a woman, she is at increased risk for obesity-related diseases. By the way, we could also identify her increased risk by using the waist circumference criteria listed previously, since her waist measurement is greater than 35 inches.

Estimating Calorie Requirements

A calorie is a unit of measurement that measures the energy contained in food. Food is our body's fuel. Eating the right amount of calories is important for maintaining a healthful weight, and eating a varied selection of nutritious foods is important for obtaining the correct complement of vitamins and minerals to maintain health. It's important to pay attention to both *what* and *how much* we eat.

Table 4.3 can be used to *approximate* your caloric requirements for *weight maintenance*. Eating fewer calories than your body requires for weight maintenance generally results in weight loss, and eating more calories than your body requires for weight maintenance should result in weight gain. Use the BMI information from the previous section to determine if you are overweight, normal weight, or underweight. Then, locate your weight category and find the column that best describes your activity level. The calorie range tells you *approximately* how many calories your body needs per pound of actual body weight. Keep in mind that this is only an estimate. More accuracy would require complex formulas or a personal assessment by a health-care professional who would take into account your gender, weight, height, age, and activity level.

> The higher the BMI (body mass index) number is, the greater the risk of developing health problems related to obesity.

Clinical experience has led me to believe that most women need about 1,600–2,000 calories per day to maintain weight, and that most

Table 4.3 Estimating Adult Caloric Requirements for Weight Maintenance

	Sedentary	Moderate Activity	Very Active
Overweight	9–11 calories/ pound	12–14 calories/ pound	15–16 calories/ pound
Normal Weight	13–14 calories/ pound	15–16 calories/ pound	17–18 calories/ pound
Underweight	14–16 calories/ pound	17–18 calories/ pound	19–22 calories/ pound

men need about 2,000–2,500 calories per day to maintain weight. Those ranges assume light to moderate activity.

Once you've estimated your calorie goals, pay close attention to what happens to your weight if you eat that level of calories. The table provides a way to estimate calorie levels for weight maintenance, but if you're gaining undesired weight on that calculated calorie range, you'll need to cut back the calories. Or, if you're losing weight unintentionally, you'll need to increase the calories.

Example 1

Leon is 5'8" (68 inches) and weighs 184 pounds. His BMI is 28, which is consistent with being overweight. He has a normal level of activity. He takes a 30-minute brisk walk at least 5 times per week. According to table 4.3, he needs 12–14 calories per pound to maintain his weight.

$184 \times 12 = 2,208$, and $184 \times 14 = 2,576$

His approximate caloric requirements are rounded to 2,200–2,575 calories per day. To lose weight, he will have to reduce his caloric intake to below that range, increase his activity and exercise, or do both.

Example 2

Lin Sue is 5'3" (63 inches) and weighs 113 pounds. Her BMI is 20, which is considered normal weight for her height. She considers herself active, as she does martial arts for an hour almost every morning and frequently takes long walks. She also rides her bicycle on weekends. According to table 4.3, she needs 17–18 calories per pound to maintain her weight.

$113 \times 17 = 1,921$, and $113 \times 18 = 2,034$

Her approximate caloric requirements are rounded to 1,900–2,000 calories per day.

Example 3

Juanita is 5'2" (62 inches) and weighs 164 pounds. Her BMI is 30, which is consistent with Grade 1 obesity. She admits that she doesn't perform any regular exercise and has a sedentary lifestyle. According to table 4.3, she needs 9–11 calories per pound to maintain her weight.

$$164 \times 9 = 1,476, \text{ and } 164 \times 11 = 1,804$$

It is important to pay attention to both *what* and *how much* we eat.

Her approximate caloric requirements are rounded to 1,500–1,800 calories per day. Since she has Grade 1 obesity, she may do well to aim at the lower end of the range. To lose weight, she'll have to reduce her caloric intake to below that range, increase her activity and exercise, or do both.

What's Next?

If you are interested in weight loss, see chapter 9 for weight loss tips and determining appropriate calories to promote a reasonable rate of weight loss. If you want to know how many grams of carbohydrate, protein, and fat you need for your estimated calorie range, see chapter 6 for carbohydrates, chapter 7 for protein, and chapter 8 for fats.

CHAPTER 5

Food Label Lingo

❦

IN THIS CHAPTER

- Reading food labels
- A word about sugar
- Listing of ingredients
- The lowdown on label terminology
- Health claims
- When food labels are not required

F ood labels—what a relief! Never has it been easier to find out what a product contains. In 1990 the Nutrition Labeling and Education Act was passed, and by 1994 food labels became mandatory for most packaged foods. One improvement offered by the new food labels was the standardization of serving sizes. In other words, the amount that is listed as "one serving" is actually set by the government. Serving sizes are now based on portions commonly eaten. In the past, the manufacturer could take one of those little lunch box–size bags of potato chips and say it had "2 servings per container." (Like any of us would actually share that bag of chips!) Then, when you looked at the calories listed on the label, you were misled. Since you were eating the whole bag, you needed to double the number of calories listed. Deceptive label claims also used to be a problem. Manufacturers could say something was "light," and we thought it meant low in calories, but in fact they may have meant light in color, texture, or weight. Those days are over. Manufacturers are now held to labeling laws developed and monitored by the Food and Drug Administration (FDA) and the United States Department of Agriculture (USDA).

Reading Food Labels

Let's look at a sample food label (figure 5.1) and break it down, item by item, to clarify its content. We'll start at the top of the label and work our way to the bottom. Some manufacturers will voluntarily include more information on their labels than is required. The sample label shows the information that is required by law to be listed.

Figure 5.1—Food Label

Nutrition Facts		
Serving Size 3/4 cup (55g)		
Servings Per Container 8		
Amount Per Serving		
Calories 200	Calories from Fat 10	
		% Daily Value*
Total Fat 1g		2%
Saturated Fat 0g		0%
Cholesterol 0mg		0%
Sodium 20mg		1%
Total Carbohydrate 45g		15%
Dietary Fiber 5g		20%
Sugars 15g		
Protein 6g		
Vitamin A 0%	•	Vitamin C 0%
Calcium 0%	•	Iron 8%

* Percent Daily Values are based on a 2,000 calorie diet. Your daily values may be higher or lower depending on your calorie needs:

	Calories	2,000	2,500
Total Fat	Less than	65g	80g
Sat. Fat	Less than	20g	25g
Cholesterol	Less than	300mg	300mg
Sodium	Less than	2400mg	2400mg
Total Carbohydrate		300g	375g
Dietary Fiber		25g	30g

Calories per gram:
Fat 9 • Carbohydrates 4 • Protein 4

Nutrition Facts

This is the title of the new food label.

Serving Size

The serving size is listed. Depending on what the food item is, the units of measure may be cups, spoons, or pieces. Be sure to notice what is defined as one serving, as this

> The Percent Daily Value numbers apply to a very specific subset of people.

may be more or less than you are actually eating. *The information contained on the rest of the label pertains to this serving size.*

In parentheses, behind the serving size, you will find the number of grams that the product weighs. Looking at our sample label, the serving size is ¼ cup. If you took ¼ cup of this product and weighed it on a food scale, it would weigh 55 g.

Weighing tip: 28 grams equals one ounce.

Servings per Container

This is how many servings are in the whole container. In our sample food label the serving size is ¼ cup, but 8 servings are in the container.

Calories

This is how many calories are in *one serving*. In our sample, 200 calories are in ¼ cup.

The label also tells you how many calories come from fat. In our sample, only 10 calories out of the 200 come from fat.

% Daily Value

These numbers, along the right side of the label, are listed in bold and have a percent sign next to them. Percent Daily Value can be confusing. This formula takes the amount of the given nutrient supplied in one serving of the product and compares it to a 2,000 calorie diet. Our sample label lists 45 g of total carbohydrate. Look at the % Daily Value column. It shows that 45 grams of carbohydrate supply 15 percent of your daily need *if you need 2,000 calories per day and you plan to have 60 percent of your calories come from carbohydrate.* In other words, the Percent Daily Value numbers apply to a very specific subset of people.

Total Fat

The number of grams of fat is listed. Be sure to look for the number that has the "g" next to it.

Saturated Fat

This tells *how much of the Total Fat* is saturated. (You do *not* add the Total Fat and the Saturated Fat together.)

Cholesterol

The milligrams of cholesterol are listed.

Sodium

The milligrams of sodium are listed.

Total Carbohydrate

By the way, fiber is not digested and does not raise your blood sugar or contribute calories.

The number of grams of total carbohydrate is listed. Due to lack of space, small packages may abbreviate this as Total Carb. This number already includes the carbohydrate supplied from dietary fiber, sugar, and other forms of carbohydrate. Starch grams are not listed separately. If you subtract the fiber grams and the sugar grams from the total carbohydrate grams, the remainder is the amount of starch or other carbohydrate contained in the product. Listing the grams of starch and other carbohydrate separately is not a requirement for food labels.

Dietary Fiber

This tells *how much of the total carbohydrate* comes from fiber. By the way, fiber is not digested and does not raise your blood sugar or contribute calories.

Sugars

This tells *how much of the total carbohydrate* comes from sugar. The number of grams of sugar listed includes both the added sugars and the naturally occurring forms of sugar.

Protein

The number of grams of protein is listed. Since individual protein requirements vary so much, the label does not provide a Percent Daily Value for protein.

Yes, that's right . . . fat has more than twice as many calories as either carbohydrate or protein!

Vitamins/Minerals

Vitamin A, Vitamin C, Calcium, and Iron are listed in terms of the Percent Daily Value. Manufacturers may choose to list other vitamins or minerals in addition to these required four.

Percent Daily Value References

The bottom portion of the label shows reference intakes for both a 2,000 and a 2,500 calorie diet. The grams of fat listed are consistent with keeping fat at or below 30 percent of the total calories. The figures show that on a 2,000 calorie diet, fat should be 65 g or less. For a 2,500 calorie diet, fat should be 80 g or less. The grams of saturated fat listed are consistent with less than 10 percent of total calories coming from saturated fat. Total carbohydrate of 300 grams per day on a 2,000 calorie diet and 375 grams on a 2,500 calorie diet are consistent with 60 percent of the diet coming from carbohydrate. Limits are set on cholesterol and sodium, and a healthful intake of fiber is promoted.

Calories per Gram Conversions

Calories per gram conversions are at the bottom of the label. It shows that one gram of fat has 9 calories, one gram of carbohydrate has 4 calories, and one gram of protein has 4 calories. (Yes, that's right . . . fat has more than twice as many calories as either carbohydrate or protein!)

Abbreviated Food Labels

Small packages have space limitations and are allowed to use an abbreviated label format. Foods that have very few of the nutrients listed on the standard label are also allowed to use a short label format.

A Word About Sugar

In case you were wondering . . . the sample label was taken off a box of Oat Bran Raisin Cereal. The cereal did not have any white sugar added to it. But wait a minute. The label says 15 g of sugar! This brings up an important concept. Both natural sugars and added sugars are lumped together on the label. The raisins in this cereal contain natural sugars. Open your refrigerator and look at the label on a milk carton. It will say something close to "Total Carbohydrate = 13 g" and "Sugar = 13 g." That's because the carbohydrate in milk is lactose, which is a *natural sugar.* All of the carbohydrate in milk is technically sugar. Relax, it's okay. Too many people use some arbitrary cut-off point for what they consider an acceptable number of sugar grams in any product. If the sugar is over such and such grams, they don't buy the product. That isn't a wise approach. It may cause you to avoid healthful foods that contain natural sugars, such as milk and fruits. A better approach is to look at the *total carbohydrate* grams, not the grams of sugar. Remember, all carbohydrates, except for fiber, turn into sugar eventually. It's best to focus on eating healthful choices with an *appropriate amount of total carbohydrate*, instead of worrying about the number of grams of sugar on the label.

> A better approach is to look at the *total carbohydrate* grams, not the grams of sugar.

Listing of Ingredients

Ingredients are listed on a package in order of descending weight. The ingredient that is present in the largest amount (by weight) is listed first; the ingredient in the second-largest amount (by weight) is listed second, and so on down the line.

The Lowdown on Label Terminology

A manufacturer cannot use certain label claims unless its product meets the government standards. The FDA and USDA regulate terms, as shown in table 5.1.

Health Claims

Manufacturers cannot lead you to believe that their product can cure every ill under the sun. Health claims can be made only if scientific studies have proven a relationship between the food and a specific disease state. Table 5.2 defines acceptable health claims.

> Health claims can be made only if the scientific studies have proven a relationship between the food and a specific disease state.

When Food Labels Are Not Required

Not all foods are legally required to have a food label. Examples include foods that are prepared at a deli or supermarket bakery, restaurant meals, and raw foods such as produce. Exchange lists and nutrition reference books can help you determine the nutrient content of foods that do not have labels. (Exchange lists are included in the appendix.) Look for cookbooks that provide nutrition breakdowns for their recipes.

Table 5.1   Label Claims

Label Claim	Legal Definition (g = grams, mg = milligrams)
Calorie Free	Less than 5 calories per serving
Low Calorie	40 calories or less per serving
Reduced or Fewer Calories	At least 25 percent fewer calories than the usual food
Fat Free	Less than ½ g of fat per serving
Saturated Fat Free	Less than ½ g of saturated fat per serving
Low Fat	3 g of fat or less per serving
Low Saturated Fat	1 g or less of saturated fat per serving
Reduced or Less Fat	At least 25 percent less fat than the usual food
Reduced or Less Saturated Fat	At least 25 percent less saturated fat than the usual food
Cholesterol Free	Less than 2 mg cholesterol *and* 2 g or less of saturated fat
Low Cholesterol	20 mg or less of cholesterol *and* 2 g or less of saturated fat
Reduced or Less Cholesterol	At least 25 percent less cholesterol *and* 2 g or less of saturated fat
Sodium Free	Less than 5 mg per serving
Very Low Sodium	35 mg or less per serving
Low Sodium	140 mg or less per serving
Reduced or Less Sodium	At least 25 percent less sodium than the usual food
High Fiber	5 g or more per serving
Good Source of Fiber	2½ g or more per serving
More or Added Fiber	At least 2½ g more than the usual food
Sugar Free	Less than ½ g per serving
Reduced Sugar	At least 25 percent less sugar than the usual food
More	Provides at least 10 percent of the daily value
High	Provides at least 20 percent of the daily value
Lean Meat	3½ oz of meat provides no more than 10 g total fat, 4 g saturated fat, and 95 mg cholesterol
Extra Lean Meat	3½ oz of meat provides no more than 5 g total fat, 2 g saturated fat, and 95 mg cholesterol

Table 5.2   Health Claims

For These Items . . .	This Claim May Be Made . . .
Foods high in calcium	May reduce the risk of osteoporosis
Foods low in fat	May reduce the risk of cancer
Foods low in saturated fat and cholesterol	May reduce the risk of heart disease
Foods high in fiber from fruits, vegetables, and grains	May reduce the risk of cancer and heart disease
Foods low in sodium	May reduce the risk of high blood pressure
Foods containing fruits and vegetables	May reduce the risk of cancer
Foods high in folic acid, taken during pregnancy	May reduce the risk of neural tube defects in infants
Foods high in potassium and low in sodium	May reduce the risk of high blood pressure and stroke

CHAPTER 6

Carbohydrates Count

❧

IN THIS CHAPTER

- What are carbohydrates?
- The importance of carbohydrate
- Dietary sources of carbohydrate
- Do all carbohydrates affect the blood sugar the same way?
- Recommended carbohydrate intakes
- Timing is everything
- Matching meals with medications
- Carbohydrate counting
- The exchange system
- Book list for carbohydrate counting and menu planning

Carbohydrates are often misunderstood in relation to diabetes. Carbohydrates do affect the blood sugar, but they do not cause diabetes. You didn't get diabetes because you ate sugar or starch. And once you have diabetes, you aren't supposed to give up carbohydrates.

Carbohydrates are digested and turned into glucose. Glucose, remember, is the body's fuel. Glucose itself isn't bad. We couldn't live without it. The blood transports glucose throughout the body, delivering this essential fuel to the awaiting cells, muscles, and organs.

Eating too much carbohydrate all at once can result in elevated blood sugar. One key to blood sugar control is carbohydrate management: eating the right amount of carbohydrate and spacing the carbohydrate throughout the day. Sometimes adjusting the diet isn't enough to keep the blood sugar level in an acceptable range, and medications may be necessary. But no matter how you treat your diabetes, carbohydrate management is a foundation strategy in controlling blood sugar levels.

What Are Carbohydrates?

Carbohydrates are one of the three main fuel sources supplied by food. (The other two are protein and fat.) Carbohydrate supplies 4 calories per gram. Carbohydrates are also referred to as carbs or carbos. You may see carbohydrate abbreviated as CHO, which is short for carbon, hydrogen, and oxygen, the building blocks of carbohydrates.

The family of carbohydrates is made up of sugars, starches, and fiber. Fiber is indigestible, so it doesn't supply calories, energy, or glucose. The smallest unit in the family of carbohydrates is a single molecule of sugar. There are three common single unit sugars (monosaccharides): glucose, fructose, and galactose (see figure 6.1).

The three single sugars can pair up to become double sugar molecules, or disaccharides (see figure 6.2). Sucrose, our common table sugar, is made of glucose plus fructose. Lactose, the natural sugar found

Figure 6.1—Monosaccharides

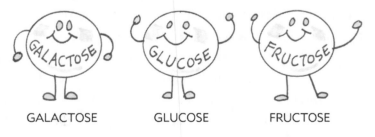

GALACTOSE   GLUCOSE   FRUCTOSE

Figure 6.2—Disaccharides

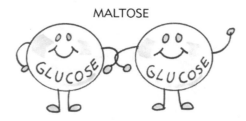

MALTOSE

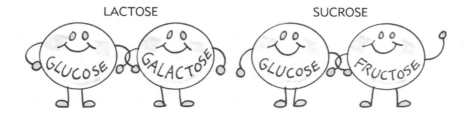

LACTOSE   SUCROSE

in milk, is made of glucose plus galactose. Maltose is the name of the sugar that is made from two molecules of glucose. Sugars are sometimes referred to as simple carbohydrates.

Starches are made of whole strands of glucose molecules connected together like links in a chain and are sometimes called complex carbohydrates (see figure 6.3).

Figure 6.3—Starches

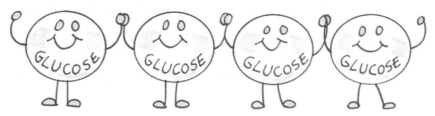

Figure 6.4—Fiber Molecule

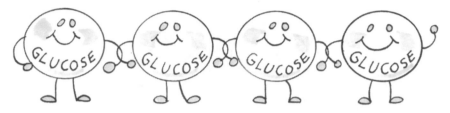

When we eat starches and sugars, the foods pass through the stomach and into the intestines where digestive enzymes break the chains into individual sugar units. Enzymes act like a pair of scissors to cut apart the links in the chain. The result is that carbohydrates, whether starches or sugars, all get digested and turned into single units of sugar. The single sugar units then get absorbed through the intestine and into the bloodstream. Fiber is also a long chain of glucose molecules (see figure 6.4), but digestive enzymes cannot break fiber into individual glucose molecules, so fiber does not get absorbed or contribute to the blood sugar.

The glucose travels through the blood and gets delivered to our tissues, cells, organs, and muscles. We need glucose to fuel our bodies just as gasoline fuels a car's engine. You can't drive a car without gasoline, and you can't operate a human body without glucose in the blood! (OK, so I'm ignoring electric cars, but you get the picture.)

The Importance of Carbohydrate

Carbohydrate digestion produces glucose, which is an important fuel source for our muscles and organs and is the preferred fuel source for the brain. Our bodies can also use proteins and fats as fuel, but in order to manage these fuels properly an adequate amount of carbohydrate has to be eaten. For instance, if too little carbohydrate is eaten, the body cannot burn fats properly.

Besides being an excellent source of energy to fuel our bodies, carbohydrate foods offer significant vitamins and minerals. Over-restricting carbohydrate foods in hopes of controlling blood sugar can result in inadequate intakes of key nutrients. If you eat the proper amount of carbohydrate, as well as include some form of regular exercise in your life, and your blood sugar is still not adequately controlled, it's time to visit your health-care provider to assess your need for other therapy options. You may need diabetes medications.

> You didn't get diabetes because you ate sugar or starch. And once you have diabetes, you aren't supposed to give up carbohydrates.

Dietary sources of carbohydrate

The main food groups that contain carbohydrate are the starches, grains, and cereal group; the fruit group; the milk and yogurt group; and the vegetable group. (See the Food pyramid in figure 6.5.)

- The *Starches, Grains, and Cereal Group* supplies important B-vitamins, iron, zinc, and fiber.

- Both the *Fruit Group* and the *Vegetable Group* offer vitamin A, vitamin C, folate, carotenoids, and fiber.

- The *Milk and Yogurt Group* supplies protein, riboflavin, calcium, magnesium, vitamin D, and vitamin B12.

Do All Carbohydrates Affect the Blood Sugar the Same Way?

It's a common question. Are all carbohydrates the same? Do various carbohydrate foods affect the blood sugar differently? What does glycemic effect mean?

Figure 6.5—Food Pyramid

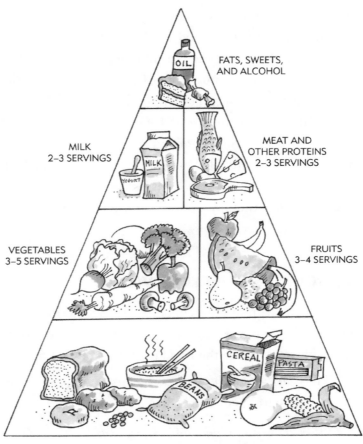

GRAINS, BEANS, AND STARCHY VEGETABLES
6–11 SERVINGS

Reproduced with permission from "The First Step in Diabetes Meal Planning."
© 1997 American Diabetes Association and American Dietetic Association.

How much carbohydrate you eat and *when* you eat it have the most influence on what your blood sugar does! Outside of that, several factors can affect the way the blood sugar responds to a meal. *Glycemic effect* describes the way a particular food or meal impacts the blood sugar. Measuring your blood sugar level at various times after a meal can assess the glycemic effect of what you ate.

Some carbohydrate foods may produce a more significant blood sugar rise than others. Liquid carbohydrates, highly processed and refined carbohydrates, and foods that are low in fiber, low in protein, and low in fat all digest quicker. Rapid digestion means that the glucose from the food enters the bloodstream within a short period of time. Too much glucose entering the blood at once may overwhelm the body's ability to process the glucose. The peak blood sugar level depends on how much total carbohydrate is eaten and how quickly the foods are digested.

Blood sugar levels usually reach their highest peak about 1–2 hours after a regular mixed meal that includes carbohydrate, protein, and a moderate amount of fat. In general, protein and fat take longer to digest than carbohydrate. Very high fat meals or very high protein meals slow down the digestion of the entire meal. Instead of the blood sugar reaching its peak 1–2 hours after the meal, the blood sugar peak can occur several hours after the meal. You may have noticed that a high-fat, high carbohydrate dinner such as pizza might show up as a high blood sugar value at bedtime. The protein and fat from the cheese and meat slow down the digestion of the dense crust, which is full of carbohydrate.

> Carbohydrate management is a foundation strategy in controlling blood sugar levels.

Factors Contributing to the Glycemic Effect of Food

- Liquids empty out of the stomach faster than solids. The carbohydrates from fruit juice and regular sodas can cause a spike in the blood sugar because they are rapidly absorbed and are concentrated in the amount of carbohydrate they contain. Use caution with juices and sweetened beverages. One cup of unsweetened apple juice, fresh-squeezed orange juice, or even grapefruit juice has the same amount of carbohydrate as one cup of regular cola.

- Foods that are *pure carbohydrate* (don't contain any protein or fat) are rapidly digested and absorbed. Fruit is pure carbohydrate. Fruit is a healthful food and should be included, but try to eat one small serving of fruit at a time. The exchange list, included in the appendix, can be used to portion fruit.

- Keep in mind that jelly beans, hard candies, and other pure sugar candies also get into the bloodstream very quickly.

- Whole grains and legumes (dried beans, split peas, and lentils) may be better tolerated than highly refined starches. These foods have a high fiber content, and fiber itself doesn't digest or turn into glucose. High-fiber foods tend to digest slower than their refined counterparts, so the resultant glucose enters the bloodstream more slowly.

- The level of food processing can make a difference. Instant mashed potatoes may raise the blood sugar more than a baked potato eaten with the skin. In general, pureed foods digest quicker than whole foods.

- Individual variation exists. Not all foods behave the same way in all people. The best way to determine how a specific meal affects your blood sugar is to *check your blood sugar!* Try checking your blood sugar 1–2 hours after a meal to monitor your blood sugar responses. Ask your health-care provider what blood sugar values are acceptable for you.

We need glucose to fuel our bodies just as gasoline fuels a car's engine.

Keep in mind that many factors, besides what you eat, can affect your blood sugar. Exercise and activity, stress, illness, and medication doses and timing can all affect your blood sugar. Be careful not to blame high blood sugar on a specific food based just on one experience. However, if a certain food produces undesirable blood sugar responses time and time again, then you may want to reconsider how much of that food you eat.

The first consideration in menu planning should be eating an appropriate amount of total carbohydrate and distributing the carbohydrate throughout the day. Diabetes medications and meals also need to be properly timed. Outside of that, the glycemic effect of food may be considered to further tighten up the blood sugar control.

Recommended Carbohydrate Intakes

Carbohydrates should provide *approximately* 50–60 percent of the total calories eaten in an average day. (See chapter 3, "Basic Nutrition Principles," for an explanation of the breakdown.)

Carbohydrate counting and the *exchange lists* are two ways of tracking the amount of carbohydrate that you eat. Once you know how many calories you should eat per day, you can use table 6.1 to decipher how many grams of carbohydrate or how many carbohydrate exchanges to include per day.

First, use chapter 4 ("Personal Profile") to estimate your calorie requirements. If you are interested in weight loss, visit chapter 9 ("Weight Matters") to find out how many calories to subtract from your calorie requirements to lose weight. It is generally not recommended for women to eat less than 1,200 calories per day or men to eat less than 1,500 calories per day unless medically supervised.

Table 6.1 provides a suggested amount of carbohydrate to eat based on your chosen calorie level.

Example 1

Jesse is aiming for 1,500 calories per day. The table shows that her carbohydrate goals are 188–225 grams per day. If she prefers to use the exchange system, she can have 13–15 carbohydrate exchanges per day. This amount will provide 50–60 percent of her 1,500 calories as carbohydrate.

Example 2

Sam is overweight. He used chapter 4 ("Personal Profile") to estimate his calorie requirements for weight maintenance. He calculated his maintenance calories to be 2,500 calories per day. He learned in chapter 9 ("Weight Matters") that by subtracting 500 calories per day, he

**Table 6.1   Providing 50–60 Percent of Calories
As Carbohydrate**

Calorie Level	Grams of Carbohydrate	Number of Carbohydrate Exchanges
1,200	150–180 g	10–12
1,300	162–195 g	11–13
1,400	175–210 g	12–14
1,500	188–225 g	13–15
1,600	200–240 g	13–16
1,700	213–255 g	14–17
1,800	225–270 g	15–18
1,900	238–285 g	16–19
2,000	250–300 g	17–20
2,100	263–315 g	18–21
2,200	275–330 g	18–22
2,300	288–345 g	19–23
2,400	300–360 g	20–24
2,500	313–375 g	21–25
2,600	325–390 g	22–26
2,700	338–405 g	23–27
2,800	350–420 g	23–28
2,900	363–435 g	24–29
3,000	375–450 g	25–30

may lose 1 pound per week. He will try to stick to 2,000 calories per day. The chart shows that he should aim for 250–300 grams of carbohydrate per day, which is the same as eating 17–20 carbohydrate exchanges per day.

Timing Is Everything

The amount of carbohydrate eaten at one meal determines the amount of glucose that ends up in the blood after the food digests. It works best to space carbohydrates throughout the day, because dumping too much glucose into the blood by overeating can challenge your body's ability to properly use the glucose and may elevate blood sugar levels.

Try to include three square meals per day. Some people find benefit in dividing their carbohydrate budget between three smaller meals and one to three snacks. Main meals should be roughly 4–6 hours apart, and snacks should be at least 2 hours after the meal. Set a schedule for meal and snack times and try to stick with it.

Example

Luke's carbohydrate goal is 270 grams per day (18 carb exchanges). The following meal patterns could be used to distribute his carbohydrates into manageable amounts.

If he doesn't want snacks, he could follow plan 1:

    Breakfast: 90 grams (6 carb exchanges)

    Lunch: 90 grams (6 carb exchanges)

    Dinner: 90 grams (6 carb exchanges)

If he wants snacks, he could follow plan 2:

    Breakfast: 75 grams (5 carb exchanges)

    Midmorning Snack: 15 grams (1 carb exchange)

    Lunch: 75 grams (5 carb exchanges)

    Afternoon Snack: 15 grams (1 carb exchange)

    Dinner: 75 grams (5 carb exchanges)

    Evening Snack: 15 grams (1 carb exchange)

Matching Meals with Medications

For individuals who take insulin or any type of pills prescribed to lower the blood sugar, it is crucial that your meal pattern be discussed with your health-care provider. Medications must be balanced with the carbohydrate content and timing of the meals. Once your medication doses are set, the effectiveness of those medications depends on your eating the same amount of carbohydrate from one day to the next. Skipping meals or eating less carbohydrate than usual can result in low blood sugar. Eating more carbohydrate than usual can result in high blood sugar.

> Over-restricting carbohydrate foods in hopes of controlling blood sugar can result in inadequate intakes of key nutrients.

Following the recommendations in this chapter may lead you to change your eating habits. *You should discuss any dietary modifications with your health-care provider before changing your diet or altering your carbohydrate intake or timing. Dietary changes may require adjustments in your medication dosages.*

Carbohydrate Counting

Carbohydrate counting offers flexibility: You have a carbohydrate budget and you get to choose how to spend those carbohydrates. Several tools can help you count carbohydrates. Packaged foods have food labels that list the grams of carbohydrate contained. Be sure to read the food label for the *serving size* and the *total carbohydrate* grams. Chapter 5 reviews the use of food labels.

For foods that do not have a food label, use reference lists. Most bookstores offer food composition books that provide a carbohydrate value for specified portions of foods. Choose a book that supplies the information you are looking for. Some carbohydrate-counting books just list the portion size and the grams of carbohydrate. Other books also provide information on calories, fat, protein, cholesterol, and sodium, which can come in handy if you need to track those values. Certain nutrition analysis books list vitamin and mineral content as well. At some point, it may become information overload!

Be wary of books that don't adequately specify the serving size. For example, if a book says the serving size is a "small muffin," it leaves the interpretation of *small* to each individual who reads the book. What is considered small by one reader may not be small to the next reader. To clear up confusion, it's best if the reference book provides serving sizes in standard measurements—for example, listing items in terms of cups, tablespoons, or weight. To use weight as a measurement, you'll need to purchase a food scale. Food scales are readily available in the houseware or kitchen supply sections of department stores. When weighing food, keep in mind that 1 ounce is equal to 28 grams of weight. And 16 ounces are in a pound.

Fast-food restaurants and many chain restaurants have product information or brochures that list nutrient information.

The Exchange System

Exchange lists can be used to track carbohydrates. One carbohydrate exchange is roughly equal to 15 grams of carbohydrate. The benefit of using the exchange system is that you count the *number of portions* that you eat instead of the *number of grams*. It boils down to easier math. Once you become familiar with the exchange portion sizes, tracking carbohydrates and planning menus becomes easier and easier.

The exchange system categorizes foods into food groups. The exchange food groups are as follows:

Starch List

Fruit List

Milk List

Vegetable List

Meat and Meat Substitute List

Fat List

The portion sizes are adjusted so that every food item on one list has a comparable amount of calories and provides similar grams of carbohydrate, protein, and fat. Thus the term *exchange*. You can choose any item on one list and exchange it for any other item on the same list, and you end up with about the same amount of calories, carbohydrate, protein, and fat. The following table summarizes the exchange system by showing the breakdown of calories, carbohydrate, protein, and fat that is found in one exchange (one portion from the list).

The three food groups that contain the most carbohydrate are the starch group, the fruit group, and the milk group. Although the milk group says that one milk exchange is equal to 12 grams of carbohydrate,

Table 6.2   The Exchange System

Exchange List	Calories	g Carbohydrate	g Protein	g Fat
Starch	80	15	3	0–1
Fruit	60	15	0	0
Skim Milk	90	12	8	0–3
Lowfat Milk	120	12	8	5
Whole Milk	150	12	8	8
Vegetable	25	5	2	0
Very Lean Meat	35	0	7	0–1
Lean Meat	55	0	7	3
Medium-Fat Meat	75	0	7	5
High-Fat Meat	100	0	7	8
Fat	45	0	0	5

a review of food labels on milk cartons will show that 1 cup of milk ranges between 12 and 16 grams of carbohydrate. I usually count the milk as 15 grams, or one carbohydrate exchange, for ease. Each of the three main carbohydrate food groups (starch, fruit, and milk) contains roughly 15 grams of carbohydrate per portion. (A "portion" refers specifically to the serving size listed on the exchange lists. See the appendix for serving sizes.) Nonstarchy vegetables contain carbohydrate, too, but not as much. One vegetable exchange provides 5 grams of carbohydrate. It would take three portions from the vegetable list to equal the amount of carbohydrate found in one portion from the starch, fruit, or milk lists. Foods from the meat list and the fat list do not contain any significant carbohydrate.

> The level of food processing can make a difference. Instant mashed potatoes may raise the blood sugar more than a baked potato eaten with the skin.

> 1 carbohydrate exchange = 1 starch exchange *or* 1 fruit exchange *or* 1 milk exchange *or* 3 vegetable exchanges

When using the exchange lists, keep in mind that the serving size listed is measured *after* the food has been cooked. In other words, ⅓ cup of *cooked* rice is equal to one exchange. It's important to use an actual measuring cup. For example: 1 cup is equal to 8 fluid ounces of milk. If you start out using measuring cups, it won't take long until you train your eye to estimate portions visually. (Though it doesn't hurt to take out that measuring cup and use it periodically. You'd be surprised how portions can grow, over time, when you serve them without using a measuring cup!)

Tip: Enlist the help of family members, housemates, and friends. Practice measuring portions. Make a game out of it. For example, cook some rice or pasta and let each person try to dish up 1 cup without using a measuring cup. This tests your ability to guesstimate. Then use a measuring cup to verify the serving sizes. Whoever scooped up the portion actually closest to 1 cup doesn't have to do the dishes!

How to Use the Exchange Lists to Count Carbohydrates

Example 1: Use the exchange lists, found in the appendix, to calculate how much carbohydrate is contained in the following sample menu.

1 cup cooked pasta   _____

½ cup unsweetened tomato sauce   _____

½ cup cooked broccoli   _____

2 meatballs   _____

green salad   _____

olive oil and balsamic vinegar dressing   _____

1 cup lowfat milk   _____

Answer: The meal contains approximately 52 grams of carbohydrate.

One cup of pasta is 2 starch exchanges, or 30 grams of carbohydrate; ½ cup unsweetened tomato sauce is 1 vegetable exchange, or 5 grams of carbohydrate (read labels on prepared pasta sauces. Carbohydrate content can vary considerably); ½ cup cooked broccoli is 1 vegetable exchange, or 5 grams of carbohydrate; meat doesn't have any carbohydrate; green salad is negligible; oil and vinegar don't have carbohydrate; 1 cup of milk is 1 milk exchange, or about 12 grams of carbohydrate (you can round the milk to 15 g if you want).

Example 2: Take a moment to plan a sample menu yourself. For this exercise, aim for a meal that provides 60 grams of carbohydrate (which is the same as 4 carbohydrate exchanges). Remember that meats and fats do not contain carbohydrate.

_____

_____

_____

_____

_____

_____

_____

_____

_____

_____

Tip: Carbohydrate counting controls the amount of starches, fruits, milk, and vegetables that you eat. One pitfall of carbohydrate counting is that it's easy for you to ignore the protein, meats, and fats that are eaten. Use sensible servings from these food groups. In general, a portion of meat should not be bigger than the palm of your hand (yes, that means the same thickness as your hand, too). Another way to portion meat is to aim for something the size of a deck of cards, which turns out to be about 3–4 ounces of meat. One to two meat portions per day are enough. Try keeping the portion of fat the same size as your thumb at each meal. Read labels for calories and grams of fat to assure that you buy the most healthful option most of the time.

> It works best to space carbohydrates throughout the day. Dumping too much glucose into the blood by overeating can challenge your body's ability to properly use the glucose.

Book List: Examples of Books Used for Carbohydrate Counting and Menu Planning

Exchange Lists for Meal Planning, by the American Diabetes Association and the American Dietetic Association, 1995.

Exchanges for All Occasions (4th edition), by M. Franz. Chronimed Publishing, 1997.

Diabetes Meal Planning Made Easy, by H. Warshaw. American Diabetes Association, 1996.

The Complete Book of Food Counts, by C. Netzer. Dell Publishing, 1998.

The Corinne T. Netzer Carbohydrate Gram Counter, by C. Netzer. Dell Publishing, 1994.

The Carbohydrate Addict's Gram Counter, by Richard and Rachel Heller. Signet, 1993.

The Diabetes Carbohydrate and Fat Gram Guide, by L. A. Holzmeister. The American Diabetes Association and the American Dietetic Association, 2000.

Calories and Carbohydrates, by B. Kraus. Signet, 2000.

Food Values of Portions Commonly Used, by J. Pennington. J. B. Lippincott Publishing, 1994.

Convenience Food Facts, by A. Monk and N. Cooper. International Diabetes Center, 1997.

Fast Food Facts (5th edition), by M. Franz. Chronimed Publishing, 1998.

Nutrition in the Fast Lane, by Franklin Publishing Inc., 1996.

Month of Meals, Volumes 1–5. Menu planners, by the American Diabetes Association, 1989, 1990, 1992, 1993, and 1994.

CHAPTER 7

Protein Provisions

❧

In This Chapter

- What are proteins?
- The importance of protein
- Dietary sources of protein
- Recommended protein intake
- Counting grams of protein
- Restricting protein for kidney disease
- Protein considerations in the vegetarian diet
- Lower-fat protein sources
- Possible health consequences related to excessive protein intake

High-protein diets versus low-protein diets. Meat-based diets versus vegetarian diets. Protein recommendations vary, depending upon which book you pick up. Popular diets come and go. What's in vogue one year can be out of fashion the next. Keep in mind that just because a diet book becomes a bestseller doesn't mean the book is factual. And to make choosing a diet approach more confusing, the scientific community doesn't always agree upon which approach is best!

Protein doesn't raise blood sugar in the same way that carbohydrate does, so why not eat less carbohydrate and more protein? This theory falls short for several reasons. First of all, carbohydrate is the body's preferred fuel source, and carbohydrate foods provide important vitamins and minerals. Diets excessive in animal protein usually provide too much cholesterol and artery-clogging saturated fat, which isn't good for the circulation or the heart. Besides that, high-protein diets may not be the best thing for the health of the kidneys because the kidneys must filter out the protein waste products.

More research is needed to firmly establish the optimal amount of protein needed to support health and well-being in the person with diabetes. Considerations include blood sugar control, weight control, blood pressure control, kidney health, and cardiovascular health. Future scientific studies could provide additional evidence that might cause us to rethink protein recommendations in the future.

The recommended daily allowance (RDA) of 0.8 grams per kilogram (g/kg) of *adult* weight is estimated to supply all protein required to meet the body's basic needs. A protein intake of 0.8 g/kg turns out to be approximately 10 percent of the total calorie requirements for a person of average weight. Most Americans are estimated to eat almost double that amount of protein, about 1.5 grams of protein per kilogram of weight, or approximately 20 percent of the total calories eaten.

Tip: A kilogram is equal to 2.2 pounds. The RDA of 0.8 grams of protein per kilogram of body weight is roughly the same as 0.36 grams of protein per pound of body weight. Either way, a calculator sure comes in handy! This chapter supplies a simple-to-use chart for estimating protein goals.

The American Diabetes Association sets protein goals for people with diabetes as 10–20 percent of total calories, the same as is recommended for the general public. Until scientific evidence proves otherwise, this recommendation makes the most sense to me, too.

What Are Proteins?

Proteins are one of the three main fuel sources supplied by food. (The other two are carbohydrate and fat.) One gram of protein supplies 4 calories.

Proteins are made of small building blocks called amino acids. Each type of protein is a unique sequence of the 20 different amino acids. In other words, meat protein and egg protein are both made of the same 20 amino acids, but the amino acids are arranged in a different order. (Just as the letters of the alphabet can be arranged to create thousands of different words, the 20 amino acids can be arranged to create a multitude of different proteins.) When we eat protein, our digestive enzymes snip the chains of amino acids apart to make the individual amino acids available for absorption into our bloodstream. Once the amino acids circulate in the blood and travel throughout the body, they become the building blocks to make our own bodily proteins.

> Keep in mind that just because a diet book becomes a bestseller doesn't mean the book is factual.

The Importance of Protein

Adequate protein intake is needed to supply the amino acids for synthesis and repair of muscle, skin, blood cells, and all vital organs. Protein is necessary to grow hair and nails, too. Microscopic, but equally reliant on amino acids for their production, are enzymes, hormones, and antibodies.

- Enzymes are crucial in keeping every aspect of the body functioning normally. They facilitate important chemical reactions. Digestive enzymes help to break down the foods that we eat into usable components.

- Hormones are messengers that relay information from one part of the body to another.

- Antibodies are our immune fighters. They battle germs and disease.

Besides the important functions already mentioned, protein is a back-up fuel source. If needed, the calories from protein foods can be burned to supply energy. However, the body prefers to burn carbohydrate for fuel and to spare the protein, to be used for the jobs discussed previously.

Dietary Sources of Protein

Protein comes from both animal products and plant foods. Examples of high-protein animal foods include meat, fish, poultry, eggs, cheese, milk, and yogurt. Plant foods contribute protein, too. Tofu, soy milk, tempeh, dried beans, split peas, nuts, and peanut butter are all examples of plant protein. You may be surprised to find out that even bread, rice, corn, pasta, oatmeal, grains, and vegetables contain protein.

Recommended Protein Intake

It's recommended that protein provide about 10–20 percent of the total calories eaten. Find your estimated calorie requirements in table 7.1. (Use chapter 4 to assess your calorie requirements for weight maintenance.) The first column is the number of grams of protein that would supply 10 percent of your total calories. The second column is the number of grams of protein needed to supply 20 percent of your total calories.

Caution: To help reduce the risk of protein deficiency, table 7.1 has been adjusted to supply a minimum of 40 grams of protein per day, no matter what calorie range you choose. Be sure to eat enough to meet the minimum RDA for protein, which is set as 0.8 grams of protein per kilogram of your body weight, per day. (That's roughly 0.36 grams of protein per pound of weight.) Eating too little protein can cause problems related to malnutrition.

High-protein diets may not be the best thing for the health of the kidneys because the kidneys must filter out the protein waste products. Diets excessive in animal protein usually provide too much cholesterol and artery-clogging saturated fats, which isn't good for circulation or the heart.

Counting Grams of Protein

Counting grams of protein on a regular basis is usually not necessary for the majority of people. (Counting carbohydrate grams, on the other hand, is an important tool in blood sugar management.)

Table 7.1 Recommended Daily Protein Intake Based on Calories Needed to Maintain Your Weight

Calorie Level	10 Percent Protein	20 Percent Protein
1,200	40 g	60 g
1,300	40 g	65 g
1,400	40 g	70 g
1,500	40 g	75 g
1,600	40 g	80 g
1,700	43 g	85 g
1,800	45 g	90 g
1,900	48 g	95 g
2,000	50 g	100 g
2,100	53 g	105 g
2,200	55 g	110 g
2,300	58 g	115 g
2,400	60 g	120 g
2,500	63 g	125 g
2,600	65 g	130 g
2,700	68 g	135 g
2,800	70 g	140 g
2,900	73 g	145 g
3,000	75 g	150 g

(Numbers are rounded to the nearest whole gram.)

Why Bother to Count Grams of Protein?

It doesn't hurt to do a spot-check once in a while to see how much protein you eat in an average day.

- If you regularly eat *less protein* than is recommended (less than 10 percent of your total calories, as listed in the previous chart, or less than the RDA of 0.8 grams of protein per kilogram of body weight, per day), you could be compromising your health. Protein is essential for many bodily functions. Along those same lines, if you eat too few total calories in the day, you will end up burning the protein foods to supply energy. The result may be that you don't have enough protein left over to supply the amino acids necessary to do the important jobs for which protein is needed.

- If you regularly eat *more protein* than is recommended (greater than 20 percent of your total calories as listed in the previous chart), you may be getting extra calories, fat, and cholesterol, which can negatively impact your health. Additional concerns related to excessive protein intake are addressed at the end of this chapter.

Where to Find Information on Protein Content

Food labels list the grams of protein contained in the specified serving size (see chapter 5). You can also use the exchange lists (included in the appendix) to count grams of protein. Measure your foods and compare your portions to the serving sizes in the exchange lists. Review the nutrient breakdown from the exchange lists (table 7.2) to see where protein turns up.

> Adequate protein intake is needed to supply the amino acids for synthesis and repair of muscle, skin, blood cells, and all vital organs.

As you can see, one starch exchange supplies about 3 grams of protein, one milk exchange supplies about 8 grams of protein, one vegetable exchange supplies about 2 grams of protein, and one meat exchange supplies about 7 grams of protein. There is no appreciable amount of protein in the fruit or fat exchanges.

Table 7.2   Using the Exchange System to Count Grams of Protein

Exchange List	Calories	g Carbohydrate	g Protein	g Fat
Starch	80	15	3	0–1
Fruit	60	15	0	0
Skim Milk	90	12	8	0–3
Lowfat Milk	120	12	8	5
Whole Milk	150	12	8	8
Vegetable	25	5	2	0
Very Lean Meat	35	0	7	0–1
Lean Meat	55	0	7	3
Medium-Fat Meat	75	0	7	5
High-Fat Meat	100	0	7	8
Fat	45	0	0	5

Here are some examples of how to use the exchange lists to count grams of protein:

- 1 ounce of meat, chicken, or fish has 7 grams of protein. That means a 4-ounce portion would equal approximately 28 grams of protein. For reference, 4 ounces of meat is a little bigger than the size of a deck of cards.

- 1 ounce of cheese has about 7 grams of protein. For reference, 1 ounce is about the size of one square inch or one sandwich slice of cheese.

- 1 egg has about 7 grams of protein.

- 1 cup (8 ounces) of milk or yogurt has about 8 grams protein.

- ½ cup pasta has about 3 grams of protein.

- 1 slice of bread has about 3 grams of protein.

- ½ cup cooked broccoli has about 2 grams of protein.

Other resources for counting protein grams include nutrition reference books and cookbooks. Look for reference books that provide information on protein content. Check for cookbooks that give a nutrient breakdown that includes the number of grams of protein in each recipe. Fast-food restaurants and many chain restaurants have product information or brochures that list nutrient information.

Restricting Protein for Kidney Disease

When protein is processed in the body, the protein waste products are removed through the kidneys. High-protein diets can speed up the filtration rate of the kidney and possibly increase the pressure in the filters of the kidney. This can be a problem if the kidney is damaged, as would be the case with diabetic kidney disease. High-protein diets can cause a damaged kidney to work too hard. There is concern that high-protein diets can cause a further decline in the health of an already damaged kidney.

Low-protein diets may slow the progression of kidney disease. However, eating too little protein can cause muscle wasting and declines in other aspects of health. Remember that protein has many important jobs. You need enough protein to sustain your health, yet not so much protein as to strain the kidneys.

The current recommendations are that if you have kidney disease, you should limit your protein intake to the minimum RDA of 0.8 grams per kilogram of your body weight, and no more. This closely correlates to eating about 10 percent of your calories from protein. (See the chart provided.) Since many people are accustomed to eating much more than the RDA for protein, sticking to the minimum RDA turns out to be a reduction in their usual protein intake. (Occasionally, doctors recommend a protein restriction of 0.6 g/kg for kidney disease. Very low protein diets should not be attempted without medical supervision.)

If you have kidney disease, counting grams of protein may become a handy tool to ensure a safe protein intake. Kidney disease may warrant other dietary restrictions, such as reducing intake of sodium, potassium, phosphorus, and fluids. These diets become more difficult to calculate and maintain, thus personalized recommendations should come from a trained professional. Seek advice from a registered dietitian.

> Counting grams of protein on a regular basis is usually not necessary for the majority of people. (Counting carbohydrate grams, on the other hand, is an important tool in blood sugar management.)

Other Things You Can Do to Protect Your Kidneys

When you are first diagnosed with type 2 diabetes, your doctor should check your urine for microalbumin. This test can detect the presence of kidney damage. Your urine should be rechecked annually to monitor your kidneys' health.

Blood sugar control is crucial in preventing kidney disease and its progression. Blood pressure control is equally important. Your doctor can work with you to achieve these goals. Certain medications called ACE-inhibitors can help control blood pressure and have a positive effect on the health of the kidneys.

Along with all the other dangers that smoking poses, it's known to be harmful to kidney health. So, if you smoke, that's another good reason to quit.

Protein Considerations in the Vegetarian Diet

Vegetarian diets can be very healthful if well planned. Vegetable-based diets tend to provide more fiber, less cholesterol, and less saturated fat than meat-based diets. For these reasons, vegetarians tend to be at lower risk for getting several diseases, including heart disease, some forms of cancer, high blood pressure, gallstones, and type 2 diabetes.

There are several types of vegetarian diets:

- Lacto-vegetarians include milk products and plant foods.

- Ovo-vegetarians include eggs and plant foods.

- Lacto-ovo vegetarians include milk products, eggs, and plant foods.

- Vegans include only plant foods and avoid all animal products.

Protein requirements can be easily met in any of the diets that include milk products and/or eggs. The vegan diet must be planned a bit more carefully to ensure adequate protein intake.

> Remember that protein has many important jobs. You need enough protein to sustain your health, yet not so much protein as to strain the kidneys.

It's important to get the full complement of amino acids (the building blocks of proteins). Animal foods contain a balance of all 20 amino acids and are sometimes referred to as "complete proteins" for that reason. Plant foods have the same amino acids, but individual plant foods may not contain balanced amounts of all 20 amino acids, so they may be referred to as "incomplete proteins." For example, grains tend to be low in an amino acid called lysine, yet they have plenty of another amino acid called methionine. Legumes (dried beans, split peas, and lentils) are high in lysine but low in methionine. It was once believed that grains and beans had to be eaten at the same meal to complement each other and form a complete protein. Now it is accepted that eating them in the same day is good enough. The focus should be on eating a well-balanced and varied diet from day to day.

Restricting all animal foods, as the vegan diet does, may result in other nutrient deficiencies. Again, careful planning can prevent problems.

The nutrients most likely to be lacking in the vegan diet are calcium, iron, zinc, vitamin D, and vitamin B12. It's important to seek out these nutrients. Here are some suggested sources:

- Vegetarian calcium sources include calcium-fortified tofu, calcium-fortified soy milk, dark green leafy vegetables, legumes (dried beans), fortified cereals or breads, almonds, and tortillas processed with lime. (By the way, lime is calcium carbonate.)

> Blood sugar control is crucial in preventing kidney disease and its progression. Blood pressure control is equally important.

- Vegetarian iron sources include enriched grains, enriched cereals, enriched breads, skins of potatoes, legumes, dark green leafy vegetables, and wheat germ. Eating vitamin C at the same time enhances absorption of the vegetable-based iron. Foods that are high in vitamin C include citrus fruits, strawberries, kiwi, cantaloupe, tomatoes, broccoli, brussels sprouts, cabbage, bell peppers, and cauliflower. (I bet some of those surprised you!)

- Vegetarian zinc sources include whole grains, wheat germ, bran, legumes, and nuts.

- Vitamin D is sometimes added to soy milk. Vitamin D can also be made in the body when the sun shines on your skin. You don't need to grease up and lie in the sun, either. Just a few minutes a day of mild exposure on your face and arms is enough. Be sure not to get too much exposure or to get burned. Excess exposure to the sun's rays can increase the risk of skin cancer.

- Vitamin B12 (also called cobalamin) sources are tough to come by if you don't use any animal products. Apparently, cooked seaweed offers some vitamin B12. Some soy beverages are fortified. Some breakfast cereals are fortified. If you don't include those products, you should take a vitamin B12 supplement.

Soy protein offers a healthful alternative to meat. Soybeans contain all of the essential amino acids. A diet rich in soy foods can actually reduce your risk of heart disease by lowering blood cholesterol levels and blood fat (triglyceride) levels. Studies have shown that eating 25 grams of protein from soy foods each day reduced the LDL ("bad cholesterol") in the blood by as much as 10 percent. (This means 25 grams of *protein*, not 25 grams of product weight. Read the food labels for the grams of protein supplied.)

> A diet rich in soy foods can actually reduce your risk of heart disease by lowering blood cholesterol levels and blood fat (triglyceride) levels.

How to Add Soy to Your Diet

Many meat-substitute products are on the market. They tend to be good sources of protein, don't have cholesterol, and are generally low in fat. Read the food labels. Lowfat is defined as 3 grams of fat per serving or 3 grams of fat per ounce. Available items include tofu, tofu burgers, tofu hot dogs, tofu bologna, soy sausages, veggie-breakfast links, soy cheeses, veggie ground round, marinated tofu cutlets, tempeh, and texturized vegetable protein (TVP) products. Go ahead, fire up the grill! Throw on some tofu burgers! Or make your own chili with veggie ground round. Give the breakfast links a try. You might be surprised at how good they are—and there's not one speck of cholesterol.

Lower-Fat Protein Sources

Compare 3 ounces of lean meat to 3 ounces of high-fat meat. They both supply about 21 grams of protein (meat has 7 grams of protein per ounce). The 3-ounce lean meat selection provides 9 grams of fat and 165 calories. The 3 ounces of high-fat meat provides 24 grams of fat and 300 calories. Do your heart a favor, and choose lean most of the time. Limiting animal fats can help to lower blood cholesterol values and helps with weight control.

The following lists can help you to choose lower-fat protein foods. It's assumed that none of these things will be fried! That would defeat the purpose of choosing a lowfat protein source.

Very Lean Meats List (0–1 gram of fat per ounce, unless portion otherwise stated)

White meat chicken or turkey (no skin)

Cornish hens, quail, pheasant (no skin)

Most types of fish, crab, lobster, scallops, clams, shrimp

Venison, ostrich, buffalo, turtle

Nonfat milk or yogurt (1 cup)

Fat-free cheeses

Nonfat or lowfat cottage cheese (¼ cup)

Egg whites (2), egg substitutes (¼ cup)

Legumes (½ cup of dried beans, split peas, or lentils)

Seitan (wheat gluten)

Soy-based meat substitutes

Lean Meats (3 grams of fat per ounce, unless portion otherwise stated)

Round steak, sirloin, flank, tenderloin, or lean ground round

Ham, Canadian bacon, pork tenderloin

Dark meat chicken or turkey (no skin)

Leg of lamb, lamb chop, lamb roast

Veal chop, veal roast

Rabbit, squab

Salmon, herring

Sardines (2), oysters (6)

Lowfat milk or yogurt (1 cup)

Lowfat soy milk (1 cup)

Reduced fat cheeses with 3 g fat/ounce

Reduced fat lunch meats or lowfat hot dogs with 3 g fat/ounce

The *high-fat* protein options to steer clear of (most of the time) would include ribs, sausage, bacon, regular hot dogs, salami, chorizo, all regular cheeses, and whole milk.

Peanut butter, seeds, and nuts are high in fat, too, but they contain a heart-healthier type of fat. (Better for your heart, but not better for your hips if you are trying to lose weight.)

Possible Health Consequences Related to Excessive Protein Intake

If you've been following a very high-protein diet or are considering increasing your protein intake to above what has been recommended in this chapter, contemplate the possible health consequences of eating too much protein.

Since many people are accustomed to eating much more than the RDA for protein, sticking to the minimum RDA turns out to be a reduction in their usual protein intake.

Over the long term, excessive protein intake has been implicated in accelerating kidney disease (for reasons explained earlier in this chapter). Very high protein diets may also cause an increase in calcium loss from the bones. Leaching calcium from the bones may weaken the bones, and this is critical for those people who are at risk for osteoporosis. High-protein diets tend to be too low in fiber. Diets excessive in animal proteins also tend to provide too much cholesterol and artery-clogging saturated fat, thus contributing to heart disease and clogging of the blood vessels. Even lean meat has cholesterol. You can cut a certain amount of fat off the meat, but you can't cut off the cholesterol. Cholesterol is in the red part, the flesh. Portion size matters.

CHAPTER 8

Focusing on Fat

❧

IN THIS CHAPTER

- What are fats?
- Types of fat
- The importance of fat
- Dietary sources of fat
- Recommended fat intake
- Counting grams of fat
- Possible health risks associated with excess fat intake
- Reducing fat intake
- Fat replacers

The health trend in the last decade or two has been to reduce dietary fat intake. Surveys show that at least eight out of ten people in the United States consume reduced-fat products. Why? Because high-fat diets have contributed to an epidemic of obesity in our country. And high-fat diets are strongly linked to heart disease, which is the number one cause of death in the United States. Plain and simple, most Americans eat too much fat.

Luckily, many reduced-fat products are available. Consumers have demanded more healthful choices, and manufacturers have responded to the tune of a billion-dollar industry that has produced nonfat or lowfat versions of dairy products, processed meats, convenience foods, salad dressings, snack foods, and even desserts. New products show up on supermarket shelves all the time. The food industry has worked hard to use ingredients that impart the qualities of fat without the calories of fat. Fat replacers are ingredients that substitute for fat. New fat replacers are being developed.

> High-fat diets are strongly linked to heart disease, which is the number one cause of death in the United States. Plain and simple, most Americans eat too much fat.

We need to be concerned not only with the *amount* of fat we eat, but also with the *type* of fat we eat. For example, when it comes to heart health, liquid oils are a more healthful choice than solid fats. But as far as body weight is concerned, all fats are created equal. A teaspoon of olive oil has about the same number of calories as a teaspoon of butter.

It may all seem a bit confusing at first, but don't give up. Take a little time to learn more about fat. What you learn may help you to develop a more healthful lifestyle.

What Are Fats?

Fats are one of the three main fuel sources supplied by food. (The other two are carbohydrate and protein.) Fats are a concentrated source of calories and, gram for gram, supply more than twice the calories of either carbohydrate or protein. Fat supplies 9 calories per gram, while carbohydrate and protein each supply 4 calories per gram.

Fats are made of building blocks called fatty acids, which are linked to a molecule of glycerol. A molecule of glycerol combined with three fatty acids is called a triglyceride. When dietary fats are eaten, they're digested into their component parts and absorbed into the body, where they're burned for fuel. If the body isn't in need of fuel, the digested fats are reassembled into triglycerides and stored in the body's fat cells.

Types of Fat

There are solid fats and liquid fats, fats from animal sources and fats from plant sources. The various fats differ in their chemical structure. The terms *saturated fat*, *monounsaturated fat*, and *polyunsaturated fat* all refer to the chemical structure of the fat. The degree of saturation depends upon the amount of hydrogen atoms that the fat chain holds. If the fat chain holds the maximum amount of hydrogen atoms, it's said to be a saturated fat. If the fat chain is missing hydrogen atoms at one position, it's called monounsaturated. If the fat chain is missing hydrogen atoms at more than one point, it's called polyunsaturated. The more saturated a fat is, the more solid it is at room temperature.

Saturated Fat

Except for seafood, animal fats are predominantly saturated. Several vegetable fats are also saturated. Molecules of saturated fat can be packed closely together. This close packing causes saturated fats to be solid at room temperature. Excessive intakes of saturated fat can raise the LDL cholesterol (the bad type of cholesterol) in the blood. Diets high in saturated fat can lead to clogged arteries and contribute to heart disease. Examples of saturated fat include butter, cheese, meat fat, chicken skin, bacon, dairy fats, coconut oil, palm oil, and palm kernel oil. Saturated fat should not exceed 7 percent of your daily calories.

Monounsaturated Fat

Monounsaturated fats are liquid at room temperature. These fats tend to be the heart-healthiest. Examples of monounsaturated fats include olive oil, olives, peanut oil, peanuts, canola oil, and avocados. But you still need to be careful not to indulge in too much of a good thing if you're watching your weight.

Polyunsaturated Fats

Polyunsaturated fats are also liquid at room temperature. Vegetable oils are rich in polyunsaturated fat. Sunflower oil, sesame oil, safflower oil, corn oil, and soybean oil are examples of polyunsaturated fat. One drawback is that if eaten in excess, polyunsaturated fats may lower your HDL (the good type of cholesterol).

> We need to be concerned not only with the *amount* of fat we eat, but also with the *type* of fat we eat. For example, when it comes to heart health, liquid oils are a more healthful choice than solid fats.

Hydrogenated Fats

Hydrogenation is the process of turning liquid oil into solid fat. Recall that the degree of saturation depends upon the amount of hydrogen atoms that the fat chain holds. Hydrogenation involves taking liquid unsaturated oil and forcing hydrogen atoms into the oil, which turns it into a solid, saturated fat. Examples of hydrogenated fats are margarine and shortening. They both started as liquid oils. The process of hydrogenation turned them into solid fats. Solid fats, including hydrogenated fats, can raise blood cholesterol levels and lead to clogged arteries.

Trans-Fatty Acids

The process of hydrogenation can cause the production of trans-fatty acids. Trans-fatty acids have an undesirable chemical structure. Excessive intake has been associated with heart disease.

Common sources of trans-fats include stick margarine and shortening. Crackers, cookies, and baked goods made with hydrogenated or partially hydrogenated vegetable oils are sources of hidden trans-fats. Trans-fatty acids also occur naturally in beef fat and butter fat.

Food labels do not require the grams of trans-fat to be listed separately. Trans-fats are lumped together on the label with the grams of saturated fat, though some manufacturers voluntarily list trans-fat grams.

Cholesterol

Cholesterol is not actually a fat. It is technically a sterol, which has a different chemical composition. Cholesterol is only found in animal products. There is no cholesterol in any plant food. We also make cholesterol in our liver. Dietary cholesterol should be limited to no more than 200 milligrams per day. See chapter 11 on heart health to learn more about cholesterol.

The Importance of Fat

Dissolved compounds in fat provide flavor and aroma to foods. Fats make foods moist and contribute to the texture of the food. That's why some of those fatty foods are so tempting! They just taste and smell so good! It may take a concerted effort not to overeat fatty foods. Fats carry with them some important vitamins and nutrients. Vitamins A, D, E, and K are all dissolved and carried in fat. These vitamins are referred to as fat-soluble vitamins. For us to absorb these important nutrients from our foods, small amounts of dietary fat must be present. When we digest the fat and absorb it into the bloodstream, the fat-soluble nutrients hitch a ride on the fat particles. You don't need to make a conscientious effort to eat added fats. The naturally occurring fats in foods usually supply ample amounts of fat to aid in the absorption of fat-soluble nutrients.

> Excessive intakes of saturated fat can raise the LDL cholesterol (the bad type of cholesterol) in the blood. Diets high in saturated fat can lead to clogged arteries and contribute to heart disease.

Fat slows down digestion time. Including some fat in a meal causes the entire meal to empty out of the stomach slower. This lends to satiety, which is just a fancy way of saying you feel satisfied for a longer period of time. Have you ever eaten a fatty meal and felt full for hours? That's because it can take four or more hours to completely digest a fatty meal.

Fat is an efficient fuel source. The body can burn dietary fats as well as stored fats for energy. When fewer calories are eaten than the body requires, fats are released from the body's fat cells and burned for fuel.

For proper growth and function, the body requires *small* amounts of fats called essential fatty acids. There are two main classes of essential fatty acids, omega-3 (alpha-linolenic acid) and omega-6 (linoleic acid). I emphasize that *small amounts* are needed because most people get far above what is essential! For example, a person who requires 2,000 calories per day would only need about 80 calories a day from essential oils. That turns out to be less than 9 grams of fat. (For reference, a teaspoon of oil has 5 grams of fat.) Most people can meet their essential fatty acid requirements with the fats that occur naturally in food without adding fat to their meals.

> Trans-fatty acids have an undesirable chemical structure. Excessive intake has been associated with heart disease.

Essential fatty acids play a role in the immune system, blood pressure regulation, heart health, vision, nerve function, healthy skin, and healthy hair. Omega-3 fats can help protect against heart disease. Fish that come from cold, deep water (salmon, tuna, herring, sardines, and mackerel) are excellent sources of omega-3 fatty acids. Plant sources of omega-3 fats include flaxseeds, flaxseed oil, walnuts, walnut oil, soybeans, soybean oil, and canola oil. Omega-6 fats are found primarily in vegetable oils, including corn, safflower, sunflower, soybean, and sesame oils.

Dietary Sources of Fat

Dietary fats occur naturally in protein foods like meats, poultry, fish, and eggs. Dairy products contain butterfat, and whole milk, cheese, cream, cream cheese, and sour cream are high in fat. Plant sources of fat include olives, avocados, coconut, nuts, and seeds.

Fats are added to foods through the use of oils, margarine, butter, mayonnaise, salad dressing, sauces, lard, and shortening. Sometimes fats are hidden in foods. You can't always see the fat. Baked goods, candies, desserts, crackers, and other snack foods often contain a lot of fat. Anything that's fried is fatty.

Recommended Fat Intake

For most people, I recommend setting fat intake at, or below, 30 percent of total calories. This is a general recommendation. Some people will require a further reduction in fat, along with overall caloric restriction and exercise, to promote weight loss.

For individuals with high cholesterol or who have atherosclerosis (clogging of the arteries), diets low in fat, particularly low in saturated fat, are often prescribed to improve heart health.

Individuals with *moderately* elevated triglycerides (a type of blood fat) and elevated VLDL (very low-density lipoprotein, a type of blood cholesterol) may best tolerate a lower carbohydrate intake and a higher fat intake, as long as the type of fat is from heart-healthy monounsaturated sources. See chapter 11 on cardiac health for more information.

Consider your weight goals and your heart-health history and use table 8.1 to find your fat gram budget. Estimate your calorie requirements (see chapter 4), then choose the column that corresponds to 25 percent, 30 percent, or 35 percent of the diet as fat.

Since saturated fat is the kind that clogs arteries, it's recommended that saturated fat not exceed 7 percent of the total calories (see table 8.2). (That 7 percent counts toward your total fat gram budget.) For most people, this means cut down! To reduce saturated fat intake, limit solid fats and animal fats.

Counting Grams of Fat
Why Bother to Count Grams of Fat?

Weight control and heart health are the two main reasons people choose to count fat grams. After all, fat is a very concentrated calorie

**Table 8.1   Recommended Daily "Total Fat"
Gram Budgets**

Calorie Level	25 Percent Fat	30 Percent Fat	35 Percent Fat
1,200	33 g	40 g	47 g
1,300	36 g	43 g	51 g
1,400	39 g	47 g	54 g
1,500	42 g	50 g	58 g
1,600	44 g	53 g	62 g
1,700	47 g	57 g	66 g
1,800	50 g	60 g	70 g
1,900	53 g	63 g	74 g
2,000	56 g	67 g	78 g
2,100	58 g	70 g	82 g
2,200	61 g	73 g	86 g
2,300	64 g	77 g	89 g
2,400	67 g	80 g	93 g
2,500	69 g	83 g	97 g
2,600	72 g	87 g	101 g
2,700	75 g	90 g	105 g
2,800	78 g	93 g	109 g
2,900	81 g	97 g	113 g
3,000	83 g	100 g	117 g

Table 8.2 Recommended Daily "Saturated Fat" Gram Budgets

Calorie Level	Daily Maximum Saturated Fat Grams (7 Percent of Total Calories)
1,200	9 g
1,300	10 g
1,400	11 g
1,500	12 g
1,600	12 g
1,700	13 g
1,800	14 g
1,900	15 g
2,000	16 g
2,100	16 g
2,200	17 g
2,300	18 g
2,400	19 g
2,500	19 g
2,600	20 g
2,700	21 g
2,800	22 g
2,900	23 g
3,000	23 g

source with more than twice as many calories per gram as carbohydrate or protein. Compare 1 cup of cooked broccoli at roughly 50 calories, to the one little teaspoon of butter on it, which contributes 45 calories! Or, 3 cups of air-popped popcorn with only 80 calories, while 1 tablespoon of oil has 135 calories. As for the heart, saturated fat, hydrogenated fat, and trans-fats can all clog blood vessels. It's not a bad idea to be familiar with counting grams of fat. You don't have to count everything, everyday, but an occasional spot check of the diet can be enlightening. Even if you decide not to count up the total grams of fat in your daily intake, it's a good idea to know what your fat gram budget should be. That way, when you look at a label or other nutrition information, you have something to compare it to. For example, if you were trying to keep your calorie intake to 1,600 calories per day, then 53 grams of fat would be your fat gram budget for the whole day (based on 30 percent of total calories coming from fat). A fast food deluxe burger with a large order of French fries has about 54 grams of fat! Once you know your fat gram budget, it's easier to make the right choices.

> Essential fatty acids play a role in the immune system, blood pressure regulation, heart health, vision, nerve function, healthy skin, and healthy hair.

How to Count Fat Grams

Food labels list the grams of total fat contained in the specified serving size. The grams of saturated fat are listed beneath the total fat. Don't add these numbers together. The saturated fat grams are already included in the total fat grams. Trans-fats are usually not listed separately. Instead they are included in the saturated fat. (Some manufacturers voluntarily show grams of trans-fats.) Some food labels will provide the grams of monounsaturated fat and polyunsaturated fat. In addition to listing the grams of fat contained in a product, the food label lists the number of calories that come from fat.

To determine the percent of total calories that come from fat, divide the calories from fat by the total calories.

Example: Using the food label provided in chapter 5, the total calories are 200 and the calories from fat are 10.

$10 \div 200 = 0.05$

To convert from decimal to percent, move the decimal 2 places to the right.

0.05 is 5 percent

The example food has 5 percent of its calories from fat.

You can also use the exchange lists (included in the appendix) to count grams of fat. Measure your foods and compare your portions to

Table 8.3   Using the Exchange System to Count Grams of Fat

Exchange List	Calories	g Carbohydrate	g Protein	g Fat
Starch	80	15	3	0–1
Fruit	60	15	0	0
Skim Milk	90	12	8	0–3
Lowfat Milk	120	12	8	5
Whole Milk	150	12	8	8
Vegetable	25	5	2	0
Very Lean Meat	35	0	7	0–1
Lean Meat	55	0	7	3
Medium-Fat Meat	75	0	7	5
High-Fat Meat	100	0	7	8
Fat	45	0	0	5

the portion sizes in the exchange lists. Review the nutrient breakdown from the exchange lists (see table 8.3) to see where fat turns up.

Examples of How to Use the Exchange Lists to Count Grams of Fat

- 1 ounce of lean meat, chicken, or fish = 3 g fat. That means a 3-ounce portion would equal 9 grams of fat. (*Tip:* A 3-ounce portion of meat is about the same size as a deck of cards.)

- Compare 3 ounces of lean meat at 9 grams of fat, to 3 ounces of high-fat meat that contains 24 grams of fat! That's quite a difference. It's no surprise that the 3-ounce portion of lean meat only provides 165 calories, whereas the 3-ounce portion of high-fat meat provides 300 calories! Now double those numbers if you eat 6 ounces! It adds up.

    3 ounces very lean meat = 3 g fat, 105 calories

    3 ounces lean meat = 9 g fat, 165 calories

    3 ounces medium-fat meat = 15 g fat, 225 calories

    3 ounces high-fat meat = 24 g fat, 300 calories

- 1 ounce of cheese has about 8 grams of fat. For reference, 1 ounce is about the size of one square inch or one sandwich slice of cheese. Cheese provides roughly 100 calories per ounce.

- 1 egg = 5 g fat

- 1 cup (8 ounces) of whole milk or whole milk yogurt = 8 g fat

- 1 teaspoon of oil, margarine, butter, or lard each = 5 g fat

- 2 whole walnuts or pecans = 5 g fat

- 6 almonds or cashews = 5 g fat

- 10 peanuts, or 2 tsp. peanut butter = 5 g fat

Other resources to count grams of fat include nutrition reference books and cookbooks. Look for reference books that list fat grams.

Check for cookbooks that give a nutrient breakdown that includes the number of grams of fat in the recipe. Many fast-food restaurants and chain restaurants have product information or brochures that list nutrient information.

Possible Health Risks Associated with Excess Fat Intake

Omega-3 fats can help protect against heart disease.

High-fat diets can lead to obesity, which increases the risk of heart disease, stroke, high blood pressure, high cholesterol, high triglycerides, arthritis, type 2 diabetes, respiratory problems, and gallstones. Diets high in saturated fat or trans-fats can lead to clogging of the arteries, regardless of your weight. High fat intake may also increase the risk of getting certain forms of cancer, namely breast cancer, colon cancer, and prostate cancer.

Reducing Fat Intake

Take a good look at your diet. If you're eating too much fat, you can take steps to reduce your fat intake. There are many ways to trim fat out of the diet.

- *Shop lowfat:* Start by shopping for nonfat and reduced-fat products. Look for the words *fat free, nonfat, reduced fat,* and *lowfat.* Read labels for fat grams (3 grams of fat per serving, or 3 grams of fat per ounce of meat or cheese indicates lowfat).

- *Cook lowfat:* Use lowfat cooking methods. Bake, broil, roast, poach, steam, grill, microwave, or boil. Don't deep-fry foods. Use a non-stick pan with cooking spray. Use lowfat recipe modifications and lowfat cookbooks.

- *Dine lowfat:* Ask the waiter for tips on healthful menu selections. Request sauces and salad dressings on the side. Don't order fried items. Limit visits to fast-food restaurants.

- *Snack lowfat:* Crunch on baked chips instead of fried chips. Use air-popped popcorn. Try lowfat crackers, pretzels, or rice cakes. Choose fresh vegetables with fat-free dip. Have a piece of fruit.

See chapter 21, "Eat Well, Be Well," for more tips on trimming out the fat.

Fat Replacers

Fat contributes to a product's moisture, texture, and mouth feel. It's easy enough to take fat out of milk and still end up with a satisfying product. It's not as easy to take all the fat out of mayonnaise, salad dressings, or cookies. Manufacturers have worked hard in test kitchens to come up with acceptable fat-free and lowfat products.

Fat replacers are ingredients that take the place of fat. Ideally, fat replacers provide the qualities of fat without the calories of fat. They can be made from carbohydrate, protein, or fat.

Carbohydrate-Based Fat Replacers

These are the most common types of fat replacers. They include modified food starch, tapioca, dextrin, maltodextrin, guar gum, xanthan gum, pectin, carrageenan (from seaweed), fiber, gels, and sugar alcohols. They're used as thickeners and stabilizers. Carbohydrate-based fat replacers are used in salad dressings, sauces, baked goods, frozen desserts, yogurts, puddings, and candies.

Fruit can also replace fat in some baked goods. For example, replacing some of the fat with applesauce provides a product that retains its moistness.

Protein-Based Fat Replacers

Protein-based fat replacers are made from modified egg protein and milk protein. Protein-based fat replacers provide a creamy texture to reduced-fat salad dressings, sour cream, cheese, spreads, margarine, and mayonnaise. They're also used in some lowfat baked goods.

Fat-Based Fat Replacers

Have you ever read a food label and seen the words *mono-* and *diglycerides?* Those are actually emulsifiers made of fat. Emulsifiers create a creamy texture and help to keep ingredients suspended and prevent separation. Fat-based fat replacers are used in reduced-fat mayonnaise, sauces, and salad dressings. Fat-based fat replacers are stable when heated.

> After all, fat has more than twice as many calories as carbohydrate or protein.

Synthetic Fats

The big push has been to create a synthetic fat with all the properties of fat and none of the calories. What if you could fry foods in a fake fat and not absorb any fat calories? Wouldn't that be perfect! Well, in 1996 the FDA approved the first synthetic oil, a product called Olestra. Olestra, also called Olean, is used to make snack foods like chips and crackers. Olestra acts like fat, because it actually *is* fat. However, the chemical structure has been modified so that our digestive enzymes can't break the fat down; therefore, it's not absorbed into the bloodstream. It's hard to tell the difference between a potato chip fried in Olestra or a regular potato chip. You even get greasy fingers handling the Olestra chip! Unfortunately, there are some drawbacks to this fat replacer. Because the fat does not digest, it can cause cramping and loose, oily stools in some people. The effect depends on how much of the product is eaten and individual response. This side effect may be an annoyance but probably doesn't pose any serious health risks. Another problem may have more nutritional significance. Important fat-soluble vitamins attach to fat particles, and that's how vitamins A, D, E, and K hitch a ride from the intestines into the bloodstream, where they're needed by the body. Other important nutrients such as carotenoids are absorbed in this same manner. In the case of Olestra, the fat-soluble vitamins hitch a ride right out of the body, since the fake fat is not absorbed. Products containing Olestra have a warning label to alert consumers to these issues, and the manufacturer adds Vitamins A, D, E, and K (but not carotenoids) to products containing Olestra.

As far as body weight is concerned, all fats are created equal. A teaspoon of olive oil has about the same number of calories as a teaspoon of butter.

Tip: When choosing lowfat products or products made with fat replacers, don't reward yourself by eating twice as much. The total calories can still add up! Some reduced-fat products have extra sugar added, so be sure to read food labels.

CHAPTER 9

Weight Matters

✍

IN THIS CHAPTER

- Excess calories add up to excess weight
- Eating a balanced diet
- Setting realistic weight loss goals
- Changing behaviors
- Using exchange lists to plan menus for specific calorie ranges
- Sample exchange system meal plans
- Weight loss programs
- Very low calorie diets
- Fad diets
- 100 tips for successful weight management
- Locating a registered dietitian in your area

Once, a patient told me that she ate a Christmas cookie the second week of December, and she figured that since she'd already blown it, she might as well wait until after the first of the year to resume her diet. It's funny how our minds work. She thought that she'd made a wrong turn, and she was ready to turn it into a full-blown detour. It's possible to work on weight loss and still include some of your favorite foods, like a cookie. What matters most is the big picture. One cookie won't make or break your weight. Your weight responds to the total amount of calories eaten and the total amount of calories burned.

At least half of all Americans are overweight or obese. Excess weight poses many health risks. Obesity increases the chance of developing numerous diseases, including:

- Type 2 diabetes
- Hypertension
- High cholesterol and high triglycerides
- Coronary heart disease
- Peripheral vascular disease
- Stroke
- Gallbladder disease
- Osteoarthritis
- Sleep apnea and respiratory problems
- Certain cancers, including endometrial, breast, prostate, and colon

Excess Calories Add Up to Excess Weight

Calories measure the amount of energy contained in food. Our bodies burn calories for fuel, just as a car burns gasoline for fuel. The calories that you consume must be fully utilized (burned for fuel), or else they will be stored for later use. Excess calories, no matter what the source, can be converted into fat by the liver. Then those fats travel through the blood to fat cells, where they hibernate until needed for fuel.

Humans get their calories from proteins, carbohydrates, fats, and alcohol. There are no calories in fiber, water, or vitamins and minerals.

Calorie Comparison

Protein has 4 calories per gram.

Carbohydrate has 4 calories per gram.

Fat has 9 calories per gram.

Alcohol has 7 calories per gram.

Notice that fat has more than twice as many calories, gram for gram, as either protein or carbohydrate. Fat is by far the most concentrated calorie source. Alcohol is a close second.

Burning Calories for Fuel

Once the calories are eaten, they can be burned during normal metabolism, daily activity, and planned exercise.

> At least half of all Americans are overweight or obese.

Metabolism is the word scientists use to describe the process of keeping a human body operating. Metabolism burns calories for heartbeats, breathing, body temperature regulation, and all of the other complex processes transpiring within our human machinery.

Our day-to-day activities use a certain amount of calories. Every time you move your body, you burn calories. The more you move about, the more calories you burn.

Planned exercise is one way to increase the number of calories you burn. Successful weight loss and ongoing weight control depend on including regular exercise in your life. In addition to the calories you burn during exercise sessions, exercise can increase the number of calories that you burn through normal metabolism. Exercise helps you to maintain muscle (and, in some cases, to build muscle) while losing body fat. Muscle cells do the best job of burning calories, so bodies with more muscle burn more calories. In this way, exercise increases the metabolic rate.

Input Versus Output

If the calories you eat are roughly equal to the calories you burn, then theoretically, you will stay about the same weight. Here's an example:

Let's say that John's body needs about 2,000 calories per day. What do you think would happen on a day that he eats 2,300 calories? The extra 300 calories would be converted to fat and stored for later. Conversely, what would happen if John ate only 1,500 calories on another day? The body would release 500 calories from its reserves to make up the deficit. If John doesn't eat enough calories, he has to use up some of his stored fat.

One pound of body fat stores roughly 3,500 calories! Ouch! To get rid of one pound of body fat requires using 3,500 calories out of storage. That won't happen in a day. Weight takes time to put on and takes time to take off. Going back to our example with John: If his body needs about 2,000 calories per day, and he continues to limit his caloric intake to 1,500 calories per day, then he'll use 500 calories from body fat stores every day. In a week he should lose one pound (500 calories per day, times 7 days in a week equals 3,500 calories). To lose ½ pound per week would require a caloric deficit of 250 calories per day.

> Successful weight loss and ongoing weight control depend on including regular exercise in your life.

Tip: Even small changes can make a difference over time. Giving up 150 calories per day saves you 54,750 calories per year! (As a perspective, 150 calories is the amount of calories in either 1 ounce of regular potato chips, or 12 ounces of regular soda.)

Tip: Talk to your health-care provider about your weight loss plans. Find out if your doctor has any specific recommendations or warnings for you.

Eating a Balanced Diet

When cutting back on calories, be sure to eat a varied and well-balanced diet. You still need the recommended amount of vitamins and minerals. The food pyramid is one tool to assist you in following a balanced diet. There is a suggested range of portions for each food group. Following the lower number within each food group helps to keep the calories low.

Figure 9.1—Food Pyramid

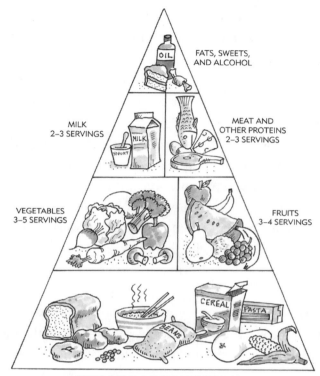

Reproduced with permission from "The First Step in Diabetes Meal Planning."
© 1997 American Diabetes Association and American Dietetic Association.

Setting Realistic Weight Loss Goals

If you're interested in losing weight, set realistic weight targets. A suggested rate of weight loss is 1–2 pounds per week. Health benefits can be realized with even modest amounts of weight loss. Losing 10–20 pounds can greatly improve blood sugar control because weight loss allows your body's insulin to work better. Health experts recommend an initial weight loss goal of 5–10 percent. For example, if you weigh 250 pounds, aim for losing 12–25 pounds. If you weigh 180 pounds, aim for losing 9–18 pounds. Then reassess. You can choose to reduce further.

Losing more than a pound per week would mean a caloric deficit of greater than 500 calories per day. Very low calorie diets can be hard to follow and they pose risks for nutritional deficiencies. I usually advise women who are working on weight loss to eat at least 1,200 calories per day, and men who are limiting their diets to eat at least 1,400 calories per day.

Tip: If you're restricting calories for weight loss and you wish to take a multivitamin, choose one that supplies 100 percent of the RDAs. Don't mega-dose!

If you want to lose more than 1 pound per week, it's best to add exercise. Burning 500 calories per day through exercise would result in using up 3,500 calories per week, thus losing one pound per week. A more realistic goal may be to burn 250 calories per day through exercise, which should result in losing ½ pound per week. Even this may be difficult for someone who has not exercised in the past or who has medical limitations. If this applies to you, don't worry. Start slowly. The goal is to do what you can safely and comfortably do and work up from there.

Tip: To promote weight loss, exercise should be included on most days of the week. Start modestly, perhaps with 10 minutes. Eventually, try to increase your activity to include 30 minutes of exercise 4–7 days per week. That can be all at once, or accumulated through 2–3 sessions in the day. *Check with your doctor and get medical advice tailored to you BEFORE you begin any new exercise program.* See chapter 10 for more tips on safe exercise.

Changing Behaviors

Sometimes people eat in response to situations or events other than hunger. For example, eating may be the behavior that follows a stressful situation, a depressed mood, or an angry moment. Eating may be linked to idle time or situations such as watching television or working at your desk. Many of us eat larger portions during social events, special occasions, or the holidays. Eating for "nonhunger" reasons is normal, if done occasionally, but making it a habit can cause weight control problems.

If you think "nonhunger" eating is a problem for you, it's important to identify what triggers your eating. Record keeping can help to pinpoint specific problem areas. Try keeping a food diary. Write down what you eat. Next to the meal or snack entry, take note of where you were at the time, what was happening around you, and how you felt. Look for patterns. Once you recognize the cue or trigger for "nonhunger" eating, you can work on making changes.

Situational Eating

Have you ever bought popcorn or snacks at the movie even though you weren't really hungry? Or have you found yourself eating at work in the middle of the afternoon, just because co-workers were congregating in the break room around a table of snacks? If so, you may be a situational eater. In other words, time and place may be situational triggers for you to eat even if you aren't hungry. Once you identify the situations that lead to "nonhunger" eating, try to plan alternative activities or develop strategies for how you'll respond to those situations in the future, *without reaching for food*. It may mean finding something else to challenge you, like taking up a craft, hobby, sport, class, or volunteer work. Try getting out of the house, taking a walk, or calling on friends. Some people can simply make a conscious decision to set limits on their eating, such as, "I won't eat in front of the television or anywhere other than a table." Try a variety of alternative activity plans or strategies and see which one works best for you.

> Very low calorie diets can be hard to follow and they pose risks for nutritional deficiencies.

Emotional Eating

Food is a pleasure and a comfort to humans. It's natural for food to play a role in our "self-nurturing." But if eating becomes a coping mechanism for emotional stress, the extra calories can contribute to weight and health problems. If you think emotional eating is a problem for you, it's important to find other ways to cope. Stress

management training and working to develop assertive communication skills can be helpful. Individual counseling, classes, workshops,
and support groups may be valuable in breaking patterns that lead to
overeating. Ask your health-care provider to help you explore your
options for controlling emotional eating.

Behavior Change Tips

- Identify what triggers "nonhunger" eating.

- Create a strategy for making a change.

- Predict challenges and devise a plan to overcome them.

- Act on your plan.

- Get support, if needed.

- Evaluate your progress.

- Don't get discouraged, and don't give up!

- Refine your plan, or make changes to your plan as needed.

- Try again until you find the right strategies for YOU!

Using Exchange Lists to Plan Menus for Specific Calorie Ranges

The exchange system categorizes food into groups. The exchange food
groups are as follows:

Starch List

Fruit List

Milk List

Vegetable List

Meat and Meat Substitute List

Fat List

The lists are set up so that you can choose any item within one list and *exchange* it for any other item on the same list, and you end up with a similar amount of calories, carbohydrate, protein, and fat. Thus the term *exchange*.

The exchange lists can be used to control portions and distribute just the carbohydrate foods throughout the day, as is done with carbohydrate counting. Or the meat and fat exchanges can be counted in addition to the carbohydrate exchanges in order to keep track of the *total amount of calories eaten*. The following menu-planning tables can be used to help you stay within your chosen calorie goal. The number of exchanges (portions) provided from each food group is listed for every calorie level. These meal plans all provide *approximately* 50 percent of the calories from carbohydrate. They supply *about* 20 percent of the calories from protein and *about* 30 percent of the calories from fat.

> Eating for "nonhunger" reasons is normal, if done occasionally, but making it a habit can cause weight control problems.

First, use chapter 4 to assess your weight maintenance calorie level. If you're interested in weight loss, subtract 250–500 calories from that number to promote a ½–1 pound per week weight loss.

You may choose from the meal plans that include milk or from the meal plans that exclude milk. Find the calorie level that you desire. Read across the row to the right of your chosen calorie level. Note the number of portions recommended from each food category. Once you know what your budget is from each food category, you can spend your budget on the foods you like. That's the beauty of it. The meal plans provide structure to control your intake but still allow flexibility for you to choose the foods you like to eat.

To determine portion sizes, see the exchange lists that are included in appendix A. Everything on each exchange list counts as one portion. For example, if you were having 3 starch exchanges at dinner, you could choose three different items in the starch list (such as ½ cup potatoes, plus ½ cup corn, plus 1 slice bread). Or you could choose to spend the budget on 3 servings of the same thing (such as 1½ cups pasta).

Sample Exchange System Meal Plans (with Milk)

Table 9.1's meal plans were developed using nonfat milk. The meat/ protein servings are assumed to be half from the lean meat list and half from the medium-fat meat list.

Sample Exchange System Meal Plans (Without Milk)

The meat/protein servings in table 9.2's meal plan are assumed to be half from the lean meat list and half from the medium-fat meat list.

Tip: If you don't drink milk, be sure to get your calcium allowances elsewhere.

The RDA for calcium (in milligrams) is:

ages 1–3 = 500 mg

ages 4–8 = 800 mg

ages 9–18 = 1,300 mg

ages 19–50 = 1,000 mg

ages 51 and over = 1,200 mg

It's important to distribute the exchanges throughout the day. Aim for three meals, or distribute food between three meals and one to three snacks. It's easier for the body to process the carbohydrate when it's distributed throughout the day, and hunger is better controlled when you're eating regularly spaced meals.

Tip: Try spacing main meals 4–6 hours apart.

Example: Lucinda has decided to follow a 1,600-calorie meal plan that includes milk to maintain her current weight. The sample daily meal plan provides her with 7 starches, 3 fruits, 3 milks, 3 vegetables, 5 meat/proteins, and 4 fats. Table 9.3 shows one possible way to distribute her exchanges. The sample menu illustrates what foods she could spend her budget on.

Table 9.1   Sample Exchange Meal Plan (with Milk)

	Starch	Fruit	Milk	Vegetable	Meat & Protein	Fat
1,200	5	3	2	2	4	3
1,300	6	3	2	2	4	3
1,400	6	3	2	2	5	4
1,500	7	3	2	3	5	4
1,600	7	3	3	3	5	4
1,700	8	3	3	3	5	5
1,800	8	3	3	4	6	5
1,900	9	3	3	4	6	5
2,000	9	4	3	5	6	6
2,100	10	4	3	5	6	6
2,200	11	4	3	5	6	7
2,300	12	4	3	5	6	7
2,400	12	4	3	5	8	8
2,500	13	4	3	5	8	8
2,600	14	4	3	5	8	9
2,700	15	4	3	5	8	9
2,800	16	4	3	5	8	10

Table 9.2   Sample Exchange Meal Plan (Without Milk)

	Starch	Fruit	Vegetable	Meat & Protein	Fat
1,200	6	3	2	5	3
1,300	7	3	2	6	3
1,400	8	3	2	6	3
1,500	8	3	3	7	3
1,600	9	3	3	7	4
1,700	10	3	3	7	4
1,800	11	3	4	7	4
1,900	12	3	4	7	5
2,000	13	3	4	7	5
2,100	13	4	4	7	6
2,200	13	4	5	8	6
2,300	14	4	5	8	7
2,400	15	4	5	8	7
2,500	16	4	5	8	7
2,600	17	4	5	8	8
2,700	18	4	5	8	8
2,800	19	4	5	8	9

Table 9.3   Sample 1,600-Calorie Meal Plan

_7_ Starches, _3_ Fruits, _3_ Milks, _3_ Vegetables, _5_ Meats, _4_ Fats

Meal	Exchanges	Sample Menu
Breakfast	_2_ Starch _1_ Fruit _1_ Milk ___ Vegetable ___ Meat _1_ Fat	2 pieces of toast (2 starch exchanges), 1 tsp. margarine (1 fat exchange), 1 small banana (1 fruit exchange), 1 cup aspartame-sweetened, fruited yogurt (1 milk exchange), herb tea (free)
Snack	___ Starch ___ Fruit _1_ Milk ___ Vegetable ___ Meat ___ Fat	1 latte (made with 8 oz nonfat milk and espresso coffee) (1 milk exchange)
Lunch	_2_ Starch _1_ Fruit ___ Milk _1_ Vegetable _2_ Meat _1_ Fat	pasta salad with: 1 cup macaroni (2 starch exchanges), ½ cup tuna (2 very lean meat exchanges), ½ cup diced tomato (1 vegetable exchange), 1 tsp. olive oil (1 fat exchange), vinegar (free) served on lettuce (insignificant), 1 small pear (1 fruit exchange); mineral water (free)
Snack	___ Starch _1_ Fruit ___ Milk ___ Vegetable ___ Meat ___ Fat	1 small orange (1 fruit exchange)
Dinner	_2_ Starch ___ Fruit _1_ Milk _2_ Vegetable _3_ Meat _2_ Fat	Stir-fry with: 1 cup broccoli (2 vegetable exchanges), 3 ounces steak (3 medium fat meat exchanges), 6 almonds (1 fat exchange), 1 tsp. canola oil (1 fat exchange), ⅔ cup rice (2 starch exchanges); 1 cup lowfat milk (1 milk exchange)
Snack	_1_ Starch ___ Fruit ___ Milk ___ Vegetable ___ Meat ___ Fat	3 cups air-popped popcorn (1 starch exchange), diet soft drink (free)

Use table 9.4 to develop your own meal plan. Practice by writing sample menus in the spaces provided.

Weight Loss Programs

There are many organized weight loss programs, some of which are very good, and others that are a waste of time, money, and effort. A few are even dangerous to your health. On the plus side, safe and effective

Table 9.4

My calorie goal is: _____

I will use the following number of exchanges (portions) from each category: _____ Starches, _____ Fruits, _____ Milks, _____ Vegetables, _____ Meats, _____ Fats

Meal	Exchanges	Sample Menu
Breakfast	___ Starch ___ Fruit ___ Milk ___ Vegetable ___ Meat ___ Fat	_____ _____ _____ _____ _____ _____
Snack	___ Starch ___ Fruit ___ Milk ___ Vegetable ___ Meat ___ Fat	_____ _____ _____ _____ _____ _____
Lunch	___ Starch ___ Fruit ___ Milk ___ Vegetable ___ Meat ___ Fat	_____ _____ _____ _____ _____ _____
Snack	___ Starch ___ Fruit ___ Milk ___ Vegetable ___ Meat ___ Fat	_____ _____ _____ _____ _____ _____
Dinner	___ Starch ___ Fruit ___ Milk ___ Vegetable ___ Meat ___ Fat	_____ _____ _____ _____ _____ _____
Snack	___ Starch ___ Fruit ___ Milk ___ Vegetable ___ Meat ___ Fat	_____ _____ _____ _____ _____ _____

weight loss programs may offer dieters an advantage of frequent contact, guidance, and support. Classes and support groups may increase your chances of success. Joining with others who are also working on weight loss and making positive lifestyle changes can be very motivating. It often helps to know that you're not alone in your efforts. Individual assessment and counseling sessions are an important part of any weight loss program.

> Time and place may be situational triggers for you to eat even if you aren't hungry.

It's important to select a program that employs trained health-care professionals who provide sound advice on health and nutrition. Watch out for programs that push their own supplements or products. If you're considering an organized weight loss program, make sure that the program can answer *yes* to all of the following questions.

- The program is staffed by qualified health professionals.

- The program encourages you to seek approval from your health-care provider to ensure that your health will not be compromised by the weight loss program.

- The program informs you of the risks and benefits of its plan.

- The program teaches you how to change the behaviors that lead to weight gain.

- The program teaches you how to eat healthfully.

- The program incorporates physical fitness and exercise.

- The program addresses strategies for long-term success, to prevent regaining weight.

- The program uses regularly available foods and doesn't rely on expensive foods that you must purchase from its organization.

- The program ensures an appropriate level of calories, protein, carbohydrates, fiber, and key vitamins and minerals.

- The program explains all costs.

Very Low Calorie Diets

Very low calorie diets (VLCDs) are usually prescribed only for people who are very overweight or who have significant medical problems as a result of excess weight. Because these programs restrict a person's diet to 800 calories per day or less, medical supervision is crucial. Without proper medical monitoring, these diets can be very dangerous. Don't try any do-it-yourself versions. VLCDs can increase your risk of developing, or worsening, gallbladder disease. Certain medical conditions prohibit the use of VLCDs. Your health-care provider can assess whether or not VLCDs are a safe approach for you.

Very low calorie diets are generally only considered when other weight loss efforts have failed. Most of these programs start with a weight loss phase, which typically lasts 3–4 months. Participants take a specially formulated, high-protein beverage as food during this phase. Some VLCD programs do allow small portions of specific foods.

> It's easier for the body to process the carbohydrate when it's distributed throughout the day, and hunger is better controlled when you're eating regularly spaced meals.

The next phase, called the "refeeding" phase, usually lasts three to six weeks. This is when solid foods are gradually reintroduced back into the diet. Emotional support and medical monitoring are important during this transition phase. Health problems can arise from "binge eating" or "excessive food restrictions" that may occur at this juncture.

The final phase, maintenance, involves behavior change education and the development of long-term diet and exercise strategies. Weekly meetings may last 18 months or more during the maintenance phase. As with any weight loss program, the importance of regular physical activity should be stressed throughout all phases.

Fad Diets

When it sounds too good to be true, it probably isn't true. There's no such thing as a pill, vitamin, or supplement that burns fat, so don't buy expensive potions or pills. "Fat burners" don't exist. If these notions were true, we wouldn't have an epidemic of obesity.

Be wary of sales pitches that promise unrealistic rates of weight loss. A pound or two of weight loss per week is all that is safely achievable.

Very low calorie diets (VLCDs) are generally only considered when other weight loss efforts have failed.

Steer clear of diets that have you eating inordinately large portions of certain foods, such as the grapefruit diet or the cabbage soup diet.

Walk away from diets that force you to eat certain foods at specific times of the day or prohibit you from combining certain food groups at the same meal. There is no scientific evidence to merit the food-combining approach.

Your astrological birth sign and your blood type have nothing to do with what foods you should or shouldn't eat.

Make sure that the diet is based on scientific evidence. Don't get hooked by anecdotal reports and personal testimonials.

Turn down diets that ask you to give up specific food groups. Each food group is important for balanced nutrition. For example, very low carbohydrate diets tend to be high in cholesterol and low in fiber and usually lack the important vitamins and minerals found in grains, starchy vegetables, fruits, and milk. High-protein diets may also cause the kidneys to work too hard at filtering out the protein waste products.

Tip: Don't take appetite-suppressant drugs or over-the-counter weight loss drugs without the approval and supervision of your health-care provider.

100 Tips for Successful Weight Management

Set realistic goals.

Take it one day at a time.

Keep a food record.

Don't use food as a reward.

Don't eat on the run.

Take small bites and savor each bite before swallowing.

Don't eat in the middle of the night (unless, of course, you're experiencing hypoglycemia).

Make an appointment with a registered dietitian.

See a counselor about behavior change.

Make crafts instead of baked goods.

Ask your family and friends to be supportive of your weight loss efforts.

Use smaller plates, cups, bowls, and glasses.

Serve food from the stove and not from serving bowls at the table.

Set your fork down in-between bites.

Eat slowly.

If hungry, have a small, lowfat snack an hour before the meal to curb your appetite.

Drink a glass of water before each meal.

Drink a glass of water before each snack.

Limit sweets and desserts.

Don't skip meals; it sets you up for overeating later.

Choose calorie-free beverages.

Don't eat for emotional reasons such as anger, depression, or stress.

Don't shop for food when you're hungry.

Don't shop for food when you're tired.

Don't overeat at holidays or celebrations.

Be patient with yourself.

Choose smaller portions of high-calorie foods and larger portions of low-calorie foods.

Keep meat portions the size of the palm of your hand, up to twice a day.

Keep fat portions the size of your thumb for each meal.

Packaged snack foods should have less than 3 grams of fat per serving.

Use a measuring cup to measure reasonable portions.

Think positive thoughts.

Take a field trip to the grocery store to look for lower-fat, more healthful options.

Use lowfat cooking methods.

Choose lean meats.

Choose nonfat and lowfat dairy products.

Read food labels to compare calorie content and fat grams.

Limit fast-food restaurant dining.

Eat vegetables at every meal.

Choose higher-fiber foods.

Don't buy tempting foods.

Limit alcohol intake.

> Obesity increases the chance of developing numerous diseases.

Let your friends and family know what your food needs are.

Include regular exercise in your life.

Take the skin off the chicken and turkey.

Don't eat fried foods.

Start your meal with a broth-based vegetable soup (choose low sodium, if appropriate).

Bring a healthful snack along when traveling or away from home.

When at work, don't eat at your desk.

Skip the butter, margarine, and mayo (or use nonfat/lowfat varieties).

Use diet soft drinks.

Share dessert when dining out.

Join a support group.

When served large portions, put half of your restaurant meal in a to-go bag before you eat.

Don't eat standing in front of the refrigerator.

Don't eat in front of the television.

Don't eat standing up.

Chew a piece of gum while preparing meals.

Brush and floss your teeth right after dinner.

Love and accept yourself.

Strive for five: Eat at least five portions per day from the fruit and vegetable groups.

> Excess calories, no matter what the source, can be converted into fat by the liver.

Reward yourself for making progress (but don't use food as the reward).

Visualize yourself losing weight.

Don't eat a larger portion just because it's a reduced-fat version.

Bring a healthful dish to parties so that you know there will be an appropriate choice available.

Drink at least 8–10 cups of fluid each day.

Weigh yourself first thing in the morning, but no more than once a week.

Snack on raw vegetables and fat-free dip.

Make a plan in advance for how you'll handle a tempting situation.

Make a list of reasons why you want to lose weight and review it often.

Avoid fad diets.

Look for the words *lowfat*, *nonfat*, or *fat-free* on the package.

Divide your food evenly throughout the day; don't eat heavy evening meals.

Don't go to sleep right after a meal.

Finish your meal with a walk instead of dessert.

Call a buddy when things get tough.

If you do eat a food that isn't a good choice, limit the portion size.

If you feel like you've fallen off the wagon, get back on.

Don't give up.

Pick up new hobbies.

Keep healthful snacks handy.

Plan your menus in advance.

Buy a lowfat cookbook.

Shop from a list; don't impulse buy.

Package and freeze leftovers for future use.

Don't strive to be a member of the clean plate club.

Wait at least 15 minutes after you finish your meal to decide if you'll have seconds.

Start your meal with a salad; use lowfat dressing.

Fill at least half of your dinner plate with vegetables.

Have fresh fruit for dessert.

Don't skip breakfast.

Eat only when you're truly hungry.

Stop eating when you're satisfied.

Don't arrive at a restaurant or party too hungry; have a small snack first.

Schedule main meals 4–6 hours apart.

Schedule snacks at least 2 hours after a main meal.

Use a small teaspoon to sample while you cook.

Politely refuse, rather than feel obligated to eat something you shouldn't.

Ask the waiter which menu selections are low in fat.

If it's a high-fat but favorite item, include it in small portions and infrequently.

Locating a Registered Dietitian in Your Area

Call 1-800-366-1655 to locate a registered dietitian near you.

CHAPTER 10

The Fitness Forum

❧

IN THIS CHAPTER

- The health benefits of exercise
- Exercise: a key treatment for type 2 diabetes
- Medical clearance
- The safety checklist
- Increasing your daily activity level
- Building your exercise routine
- Caution! When to stop exercising
- Strategies for staying with it
- Tracking your progress

Regular exercise is one of the best things you can do for your overall health, and it's an essential part of taking care of your diabetes. Perhaps you already exercise regularly. If so, that's great. Keep it up! But if you fall into the category of the well intentioned who mean to exercise but don't actually get around to doing it, then I hope this chapter will give you a jump-start.

Exercise should be a pleasant experience. It doesn't have to leave you huffing and puffing. It shouldn't be painful. You don't have to work yourself into a dripping sweat, and you don't have to wear spandex for it to count! You just have to move your body. Find activities that appeal to you. Then plan exercise into your day. How many of you have put exercise on the list of things to do, but by the end of the day exercise has somehow been bumped to the bottom of the list and there just wasn't time to fit everything in? (It's happened to me, too.) Exercise is often easier said than done. You simply have to make it a priority. You're worth it.

The Health Benefits of Exercise

- Exercise helps to lower the blood sugar.

- Exercise helps insulin to work better.

- Exercise helps with weight control.

- Exercise strengthens the heart and lungs.

- Exercise helps to lower the bad types of blood cholesterol.

- Exercise helps to lower triglycerides (blood fats).

- Exercise helps to raise the HDL cholesterol (the good type of blood cholesterol).

- Exercise improves circulation.

- Exercise helps to lower blood pressure.

- Exercise reduces your risk of heart disease and stroke.

- Exercise improves strength and endurance.

- Exercise helps to tone and build muscles.

- Exercise improves bone density and reduces the risk of osteoporosis.

- Exercise relieves stress.

- Exercise improves sleep.

- Exercise provides entertainment and socialization.

- Exercise makes you feel good about yourself!

- Exercise might help to prevent type 2 diabetes in those at risk for developing diabetes.

- Exercise improves overall health and well-being, which means you might spend less money on medical care.

Figure 10.1—Exercise Prescription

Rx **Prescription for Health**	*Your Name Here* *Today's Date*
Rx number 1 *Increase Your Daily Activity Level*	Directions *Begin today.*
Rx number 2 *Exercise Regularly*	*Start modestly and increase as tolerated.*
MD Signature: *Check with your doctor. Make sure that your planned exercise routine is safe for you to begin.*	

Can you think of any other single intervention that can do so much? Exercise is a prescription for your good health. Start modestly. You don't need to go out and run a marathon. You can build your exercise routine little by little. The most important step is getting started!

Exercise: A Key Treatment for Type 2 Diabetes

Blood sugar control: Exercise helps to lower blood sugar. When you exercise, your own insulin works more efficiently to move the glucose out of the bloodstream and into the muscles, where the sugar is burned as fuel. An exercising muscle uses more sugar than a resting muscle.

Tip: Find out how exercise affects your blood sugar. Test your blood sugar before exercising. Then do some exercise (for example, take a walk), and then test your blood sugar again. The results may surprise and motivate you!

Weight control: Excess body fat increases insulin resistance and worsens type 2 diabetes. (Insulin resistance means that your pancreas makes

> Exercise should be a pleasant experience. . . . You don't have to work yourself into a dripping sweat. And you don't have to wear spandex for it to count!

insulin, but that the insulin doesn't work very well.) Exercise burns fat, which helps with weight control. Achieving and maintaining a reasonable weight is a key to preventing and treating type 2 diabetes. Even losing 5 to 10 pounds can improve insulin action.

Medical Clearance

Exercise helps to lower your blood sugar. When you exercise, your own insulin works more efficiently to move the glucose out of the bloodstream and into the muscles, where the sugar is burned as fuel.

Before starting an exercise regimen, get your doctor's approval. Having a medical check-up can ensure that you don't have any complications that could be worsened by exercise. Your doctor can advise you of specific exercise guidelines and limitations if you have diabetes-related complications.

You may need an exercise stress test to make sure that it's safe for you to start a new exercise routine. During an exercise stress test, your heart is monitored while you ride a stationary bike or walk on a treadmill. Other tests may be performed at your doctor's discretion.

An exercise stress test is recommended for:

- Anyone who is over 35 years old
- Anyone who has had type 2 diabetes for more than 10 years
- Anyone with heart disease
- Anyone with risk factors for developing heart disease
- Anyone with diabetic eye disease or kidney disease
- Anyone with blood vessel disease or circulatory problems
- Anyone with diabetic nerve disease

Once you have been evaluated, your exercise routine can be tailored to offer you the benefits of exercise, without putting you at undue risk for problems.

The Safety Checklist

Safety first. Take precautions to ensure that you can safely enjoy your workout. It's important to get off on the right foot. A little prevention goes a long way!

Test Your Blood Sugar

If you take medications that lower your blood sugar, it's important to test your blood sugar before and after exercise to find out how it responds to your exercise regimen. Significant amounts of exercise can have a blood sugar–lowering effect for several hours after the workout. Check your blood sugar any time you feel the symptoms of low blood sugar. If you have very long exercise sessions, you may need to stop and check your blood sugar during your workout. If you find that exercise causes low blood sugar, then ask your doctor about getting your medication doses adjusted. Medication doses often need to be reduced, and sometimes medications can be eliminated once exercise habits become established.

Wear the Proper Attire

Dress appropriately for the type of exercise that you have chosen. Dress for the weather and wear safety gear (such as helmets, goggles, gloves, and pads) for sports and activities that warrant it.

Avoid Exercising in Temperature Extremes

Don't exercise when it's extremely hot, humid, or cold.

Carry Medical Identification

In case you are injured and need medical assistance, it makes sense to wear a medical alert bracelet, necklace, or watchband clip that says you have diabetes.

Stay Hydrated

Drink plenty of water. Exercise increases your fluid needs. For long exercise sessions, carry water with you and drink throughout your workout. Sugary beverages such as sodas, sports drinks, and even natural juices can drive the blood sugar up. The best beverage to keep yourself hydrated before, during, and after exercise is good old H_2O (water)!

Tip: Alcoholic beverages don't count toward fluid replacement. The combination of alcohol and exercise can cause serious low blood sugar reactions in people who take insulin or certain diabetes pills.

> Significant amounts of exercise can have a blood sugar–lowering effect for several hours after the workout. Check your blood sugar any time you feel symptoms of low blood sugar.

Carry Carbohydrates

If you take medications that can cause low blood sugar, carry some form of carbohydrate that can be eaten to bring your blood sugar up quickly. Fruit juice, fresh fruit, dried fruit, glucose tablets, or hard candies are examples of appropriate treatment choices for low blood sugar. For more information on treating low blood sugar, see chapter 17.

If you don't take medications that can cause low blood sugar, then you're not at risk for hypoglycemia, and a pre-exercise snack is probably not needed. In fact, if you snack unnecessarily, you may end up just burning your snack for fuel instead of burning unwanted body-fat stores.

Be Kind to Your Feet

Wear clean, absorbent socks that don't bunch up. Wear comfortable, well-fitting shoes that are designed for your particular activity. Inspect your feet daily. This is especially important if you have reduced sensation in your feet or circulatory problems. Watch for blisters, sores, cracks, or redness. Promptly report any abnormalities to your doctor.

Figure 10.2—Armchair Exercises

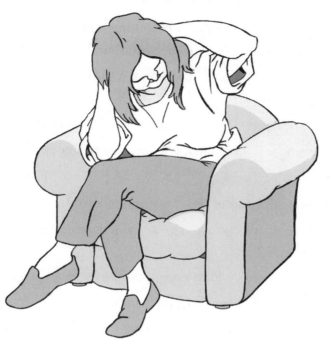

If you have difficulty seeing your feet, use a hand-held mirror or ask someone else to inspect your feet for you.

If you have decreased sensation in your feet from nerve damage, then you must select exercises that don't put your feet at risk for injury. Don't choose running, jogging, stair climbing, treadmill, or excessive amounts of walking, as these exercises can lead to injury to the soft tissue and to the bones in the feet. Good choices are swimming and bicycling. Exercises that are done while seated are also appropriate (see figure 10.2).

Sick Days

Don't exercise when you are ill, feverish, or if you have extremely high blood sugar levels.

Increasing Your Daily Activity Level

Start by taking small steps toward becoming more active. There are many ways to add activity to your daily routine. Here are a few ideas:

- Do stretching exercises while you watch the news or any favorite program.
- Do sit-ups or leg lifts during all television commercial breaks.
- Limit the amount of time that you spend in front of the television.
- Take the dog for a walk.
- Take the stairs instead of the elevator or escalator.
- Get off the elevator one flight away from your destination and walk up the last flight.
- Use your bicycle to do local errands, or go by foot.
- Park your car at the far side of the parking lot.
- Get off the bus one stop away from your destination and walk the rest of the way.
- Put the home exercise equipment in a location that will encourage its use.
- Take an after-dinner walk with family or friends.
- When at work, spend part of your lunch hour taking a walk.
- Take a walk around the perimeter of the mall before you begin shopping.
- Schedule family time doing something active.

Building Your Exercise Routine
Choose Your Activities

What sounds good to you? Walking, riding a stationary bike, ballroom dancing, a water aerobics class, tennis, golf, or an armchair aerobics video? It's up to you. You have to choose something that you like or else you'll never stick with it. (Personally, I'm not interested in running unless someone mean is chasing me. So, running isn't on my agenda.) It's also important to pick something that you're physically capable of doing without injuring yourself. Choose a couple of different activities, and then rotate what you do. That way, you're less likely to get bored with your exercise regimen.

Types of Exercise

Aerobic exercise: Aerobic exercise involves repetitious contractions of the large muscle groups, such as your arms and legs. Aerobic exercises are the type most beneficial for blood sugar control, weight control, and heart health. Examples of aerobic activities include walking, water aerobics, bike riding, swimming, dancing, rowing, running, tennis, skating, skiing, jumping rope, racquetball, jogging, stair climbing, volleyball, basketball, calisthenics, soccer, and aerobics classes or videos.

> For long exercise sessions, carry water with you and drink throughout your workout. Sugary beverages such as sodas, sports drinks, and even natural juices can drive the blood sugar up.

Resistance exercise: Resistance exercises are also known as conditioning exercises, or anaerobic activities. An example of resistance exercise is weight lifting. That includes the use of hand weights, dumbbells, and the weight machines at the gym. Push-ups and sit-ups are also forms of resistance exercise. Resistance exercises help to tone and build muscles. Resistance exercises can help maintain lean muscle while you work on losing unwanted body fat. Even the elderly can benefit from a weight-training program that utilizes light weights to help maintain muscle strength.

Caution: People with diabetes-related complications such as retinopathy (eye damage), nephropathy (kidney damage), high blood pressure, or heart disease may be advised against doing certain resistance exercises. Activities that cause straining or bearing down can cause dangerous increases in pressure that can further damage eyes, kidneys, and the heart. Check with your doctor for advice on whether it's safe for you to do resistance exercises.

Flexibility exercise: Flexibility exercises help to keep you limber. They also reduce muscle tension. Stretching, ballet, yoga, and martial arts are examples of exercises that can increase flexibility.

Frequency, Intensity, and Duration

There are three main components to your exercise routine: how much, how hard, and how long to exercise. You have to gradually work up to your optimal routine. If you don't currently do any exercise at all, you might start with 5- to 10-minute exercise sessions a couple of days per week. As your body gets used to the increased activity, you can increase your workouts by 5 minutes. In a few weeks you may be up to 15 minutes, then eventually 20, 25, and 30 minutes. You can also increase the number of days per week that you exercise. Be realistic. Don't get discouraged. Don't give up. Just gradually add to your routine.

> If you take medications that can cause low blood sugar, carry some form of carbohydrate that can be eaten to bring your blood sugar up quickly.

Frequency

Frequency refers to how often to exercise. For cardiac fitness and blood sugar control you should exercise at least 3–4 days per week, preferably every other day. For weight loss, exercise should be done 5–7 days per week.

Intensity

Intensity refers to how hard you should push yourself. You'll be the best judge of what's safe and comfortable for you. Keep yourself moving as best you can, but if you feel like you need to stop for a breather, take a short rest before continuing. You shouldn't push yourself into a state of breathlessness. You should be able to carry on a conversation without huffing and puffing. However, if you can sing the national anthem, then you probably aren't pushing yourself hard enough! Basically, you should be able to feel that your pulse and breathing are up a bit from your usual resting state. Forget the old saying "no pain, no gain." That's nonsense.

One way to measure the intensity of your workout is to take your pulse. Put your finger on one of the main blood vessels located on your neck (the arteries that lie on either side of your Adam's apple). Feel for your pulse. (You can also use the inside of your wrist to check your pulse.) Count the number of times that your heart beats in 15 seconds, then use table 10.1 as a general guideline to see what your target heart rate should be, based on your age.

Table 10.1 Target Heart Rate

Age	Target Heart Rate (number of beats in 15 seconds)
20	25–38
25	24–37
30	24–36
35	23–35
40	23–34
45	22–33
50	21–32
55	21–31
60	20–30
65	19–29
70	19–28

Tip: The number of beats in the previous chart equal 50–75 percent of maximal heart rate. (Maximal heart rate is calculated as 220 minus your age.) While some people may be able to safely exercise at intensities higher than this, other individuals may need to exercise at lower intensities. Ask your doctor if you have medical reasons that warrant a lower intensity workout.

Caution: A type of nerve damage called cardiac autonomic neuropathy can cause serious exercise-related complications. It can also prevent the heart rate from increasing normally. If your doctor has diagnosed you with this disorder, you should not try to measure your target heart rate. Instead, you should follow your doctor's advice regarding exercise to ensure a safe exercise routine.

> At the end of each month (or week, whatever you choose) give yourself a reward for achieving your exercise goals. (No, chocolate cake isn't the best reward!)

Duration

Duration addresses how long your workout should last. There should always be a 5- to 10-minute warm-up period before the main exercise session, and you should finish with a 5- to 10-minute cool-down period. The main exercise session, when you reach target heart rate, should ultimately be sustained for 20–45 minutes. But you can start with less and work up to that goal slowly. As your body becomes more accustomed to exercise, you'll find that your stamina improves and you can increase the time of your session. Table 10.2 can be used to help you slowly increase the duration of your workouts.

The Surgeon General's report on Physical Activity and Health encourages that we *accumulate* 30 minutes of physical activity per day, most days of the week. If you don't feel as if you can do 30 minutes all at once, then try for two 15-minute sessions in the same day. Or, aim for three 10-minute sessions per day. It all adds up to better health.

Warming Up and Cooling Down

All workouts should include a 5- to 10-minute warm-up period at the beginning and a 5- to 10-minute cool-down period at the end. This helps

Table 10.2   Increasing the Duration of Your Workout

Warm Up	Exercise Session	Cool Down
5–10 min.	5 min.	5–10 min.
5–10 min.	10 min.	5–10 min.
5–10 min.	15 min.	5–10 min.
5–10 min.	20 min.	5–10 min.
5–10 min.	25 min.	5–10 min.
5–10 min.	30 min.	5–10 min.
5–10 min.	35 min.	5–10 min.
5–10 min.	40 min.	5–10 min.
5–10 min.	45 min.	5–10 min.

to prevent injury. To warm up, walk or start your aerobic activity at a slow pace and with low intensity. This gets your heart, lungs, and muscles ready to go. Then you can gradually increase the pace for your exercise session. When it comes time to finish, slow down again. Do your activities at a slow pace and easy intensity while your breathing and heart rate come back to normal. You can also do some light stretching during the warm-up and cool-down phases. Stretching can help to prevent muscle stiffness.

Caution! When to Stop Exercising

You should immediately stop exercising and seek medical attention if you have any of the following symptoms:

- Chest pain
- Pain or tightness that radiates down your arms or in your neck, back, shoulders, or jaw

- Significant shortness of breath

- Lightheadedness or dizziness

- Irregular heart rhythms

- Significant pain in your joints or muscles

- Foot injury

- Short-term changes in your vision

- Any other symptom that *you* feel is serious. Listen to your body.

Strategies for Staying with It

Once you have established an exercise routine, it's important to stick to it! Motivation is a renewable resource! Here are a few tips to help keep you motivated:

- *Set up a reward system.* At the end of each month (or week, whatever you choose) give yourself a reward for achieving your exercise goals. (No, chocolate cake isn't the best reward!) Rewards should be nonfood items. How about a new item of clothing, flowers, a dinner out, a trip to the movies, tickets to the ballgame, or something else that's special to you.

- *Set up a buddy system.* If your friend is in the park waiting for you to show up for your scheduled walk, you're less likely to blow it off. Besides, it's nice to visit while you exercise.

- *Join an exercise class.* There's something very motivating about being surrounded by a group of people who are working out together. Find an exercise class with people whose exercise abilities match your own.

- *Join a club.* Walking clubs, bird-watching groups, bicycling clubs, and so on, are all good ways to get exercise and see interesting sights at the same time. You'll probably even make new friends.

- *Exercise videos.* Check out an exercise video from the local library, or buy your own copy. Plug it into the VCR and exercise in the privacy of your home. It's convenient and you can do it whatever time of day works best for you. If you don't have a VCR, tune in to a television exercise program.

- *Join a gym.* Gyms offer a variety of exercise options, classes, and equipment. A trained staff member will usually show you how to use the equipment safely and can help you plan an exercise routine.

> Regular exercise is one of the best things you can do for your overall health, and it's an essential part of taking care of your diabetes.

- *Take advantage of community pools.* Call your local high schools, colleges, and recreational centers to find out if their pools are open to the public. Hours are often set aside for lap swimming. Sometimes water aerobics classes are held at community pools.

- *Structure family time around physical activity.* Set aside some time every week for family members to do something active together. Take a hike, a bike ride, a stroll through the zoo; shoot a basketball; throw a Frisbee in the park; canoe or kayak on the lake; go cross-country skiing, snowshoeing, sightseeing, or anything else that sounds fun to you. Spending active time together is good for everyone's health. You will also create lasting memories.

- *Track your progress.* Keep an exercise diary (see figure 10.3). Record your exercise sessions. Keep track of other data that's important to you and shows your progress, such as improved blood sugar levels and changes in weight.

Figure 10.3—Activity Record

Date/Time	Type of Exercise	Minutes Exercised	Comments

CHAPTER 11

Cardiac Health: Getting to the Heart of the Matter

❧

IN THIS CHAPTER

- Cholesterol and fats in the blood
- The risk factors for heart disease
- Tackling the risk factors
- Cholesterol and fats in food
- Soluble fiber
- Summary of heart-healthy dietary tips

In a book about nutrition and diabetes, why is it so important to devote a chapter to heart health? There are several reasons. Foremost is the unfortunate fact that heart disease is the number one cause of death in the United States. We all need to be concerned. Having diabetes even further increases your risk of developing heart disease. Here's a sobering statistic: As many as two-thirds of people with diabetes die of some form of heart or blood vessel disease. Fortunately, implementing some key self-care strategies can significantly minimize your risk.

Cholesterol and Fats in the Blood

The cholesterol and fats in the blood are called *lipids*. Having high levels of cholesterol and blood fats is called *hyperlipidemia*. The National Heart,

Lung, and Blood Institute (of the National Institutes of Health) has an expert panel that has been assigned to come up with recommendations for detecting, evaluating, and treating hyperlipidemia. The National Cholesterol Education Program (NCEP) released its updated recommendations in May 2001. The new guidelines call for stricter control of blood cholesterol levels and more aggressive treatment for people who are at increased risk for heart disease.

The general adult population should have their lipid levels assessed every five years. If you have diabetes, you should have your lipids checked every year. (If your lipids are in the target range, then checking every other year is fine.) The blood test should include total cholesterol, LDL cholesterol, HDL cholesterol, and triglyceride levels.

> As many as two-thirds of people with diabetes die of some form of heart or blood vessel disease. Fortunately, implementing some key self-care strategies can significantly minimize your risk.

Total Cholesterol

Cholesterol isn't technically a type of fat. It's a sterol, which is a waxy, fat-like substance. Cholesterol is made in the body, by the liver, and has several important functions. Cholesterol is used to manufacture bile, which is a digestive juice. Cholesterol is needed to produce hormones and to make vitamin D. Cell membranes require cholesterol to work properly. Despite its positive attributes, cholesterol has its down side. As cholesterol travels through the bloodstream, it can cause a waxy build-up on the inner walls of the blood vessels, similar to the way sludge builds up in your home plumbing pipes.

When you get your blood lipids tested, the *total cholesterol* number is calculated from the different types of cholesterol and fat in the blood. Compare your total cholesterol value to table 11.1.

LDL Cholesterol

Elevated LDL cholesterol is associated with an increased risk for heart disease (see table 11.2 for classifications). LDL cholesterol is often

Table 11.1   Total Cholesterol Classifications (mg/dl)

Desirable	under 200
Borderline High	200–239
High	240 and higher

referred to as the "bad cholesterol." It's the type of cholesterol that's deposited in the blood vessels. The sludge build-up is called plaque and can lead to hardening of the arteries, also known as atherosclerosis. People with type 2 diabetes are more likely to have small, dense LDL particles, which are even worse than normal LDL particles.

HDL Cholesterol

HDL cholesterol is often referred to as the "good cholesterol." It functions to clean out the cholesterol that has already been deposited in the arteries. Low HDL cholesterol levels are associated with an increased risk for heart disease. High HDL cholesterol levels are protective against heart disease. (See table 11.3 for classifications.)

Table 11.2   LDL Cholesterol Classifications (mg/dl)

Optimal	under 100
Near Optimal	100–129
Borderline High	130–159
High	160–189
Very High	190 or higher

Table 11.3   HDL Cholesterol Classifications (mg/dl)

Desirable	over 40
Optimal	60 or higher

(The American Diabetes Association recommends HDL levels greater than 45 in men, and greater than 55 in women.)

Remember that HDL is good. Picture it as the Boy Scout troop that cleans up the graffiti on the artery walls. LDL, the bad cholesterol, lays down the graffiti, and HDL cleans it up. The more HDL, the better the cleanup goes.

Triglycerides

Triglycerides are the fats that circulate in the blood (see table 11.4 for classifications). A high triglyceride level is associated with an increased risk for heart disease. Triglycerides can come from dietary fats that we eat, but our bodies can also make triglycerides out of extra calories consumed from any source. If you eat more calories than your body requires, the extra calories can be converted to triglycerides and stored in fat cells.

Table 11.4   Triglycerides Classifications (mg/dl)

Desirable	under 150
Borderline High	150–199
High	200–499
Very High	500 and higher

Summing It Up

- Your total cholesterol should be under 200.

- Your LDL cholesterol should be under 100.

- Your HDL cholesterol should be over 40.

- Your triglycerides should be under 150.

The Risk Factors for Heart Disease

Smoking

Hypertension (high blood pressure)

Hyperlipidemia (high cholesterol or high triglycerides)

Low HDL cholesterol (levels below 40 mg/dl)

Elevated levels of homocysteine in the blood

Diabetes mellitus

Obesity

Physical inactivity

Family history of heart disease

Advancing age: men older than 45 years, women older than 55 years

As cholesterol travels through the bloodstream, it can cause a waxy build-up on the inner walls of the blood vessels, similar to the way sludge builds up in your home plumbing pipes.

Tackling the Risk Factors

You can do something about most of these risk factors! The only two risk factors you can't control are your family history and your age. (You can't pick which family you're born into, and lying about your age doesn't reduce your risk for heart disease!)

The first step in protecting yourself from heart disease is to make an appointment with your doctor and get a physical exam. Have your blood lipid levels tested. Discuss your personal risk factors with your health-care provider. The risk for heart disease is much higher when you have multiple risk factors.

Let's take a look at the risk factors that are modifiable and outline some steps that you can take to reduce your risk of heart disease.

Smoking

I know it's much easier said than done, but quit. Your risk goes up with the number of cigarettes you smoke each day. Start by cutting back, but ultimately, you should quit completely. Smoking is a major risk factor for heart disease and stroke. It also raises blood pressure; causes lung diseases, including cancer and emphysema; lowers the HDL (good type of cholesterol); and impairs wound healing. Breathing second-hand smoke can cause the same problems. Speak to your doctor about getting help with smoking cessation.

Hypertension

Normal blood pressure is 120/80. In general, a blood pressure of 140/90 is considered high—that means if *either* the systolic (upper number) is 140 or higher *and/or* the diastolic (lower number) is 90 or higher. People with multiple risk factors or who have diabetes should strive for even lower values, less than 130/80. Your physician can choose a safe target for you.

> Picture HDL as the Boy Scout troop that cleans up the graffiti on the artery walls. LDL, the bad cholesterol, lays down the graffiti, and HDL cleans it up.

Strategies to lower blood pressure include weight control, regular exercise, limiting dietary salt intake, restricting alcohol intake, and smoking cessation. Some studies suggest that adequate intake of potassium, calcium, and magnesium helps to regulate blood pressure, but more studies are needed for conclusive proof. Hypertension must be controlled. If you've done everything in your power to achieve normal blood pressure and it still remains elevated, you should speak to your doctor about adding blood pressure medications. For more information on blood pressure, see chapter 12.

Hyperlipidemia

When you have high levels of cholesterol or fat in your blood it's called hyperlipidemia. Eating too much saturated fat, hydrogenated fat, trans-fat, or dietary cholesterol can raise LDL ("bad" cholesterol) levels. Overuse of oils, fats, and alcohol can raise triglyceride levels, as can a diet that is excessive in sugars and refined carbohydrates. Lifestyle changes can improve blood lipid levels. Here's what you can do:

- Reduce your intake of saturated, hydrogenated, and trans-fats. Solid fats and animal fats are the primary culprits in raising LDL cholesterol values.

- Eat more soluble fiber to help lower LDL cholesterol levels. Soluble fiber is found in oats, legumes, and many fruits and vegetables. (See chapter 18 for more fiber facts.)

- Eat more fresh fish. Omega-3 fatty acid, a special type of fat that's found in fish, is shown to lower triglycerides as well as prevent blood clots.

- Control your weight and your blood sugar. Both obesity and poorly controlled diabetes can worsen hyperlipidemia.

- Include exercise in your lifestyle.

If your liver makes too much cholesterol or your body doesn't process fats correctly, then you can end up with high blood cholesterol or high triglycerides even with a reasonable diet. Hyperlipidemia is often inherited. If therapeutic lifestyle changes (TLC) don't adequately control your lipid levels, you'll likely require medications.

Low HDL Cholesterol

HDL cholesterol levels less than 40 mg/dl count as a risk factor for heart disease. Unfortunately, there's no food you can eat that provides this "good" type of cholesterol. HDL is made in your body. Exercise helps to improve HDL levels, as does weight loss (if you're overweight).

Studies show that a *modest* intake of alcohol may improve HDL levels. Modest means one to two drinks per day (one for a woman, two for a man). This is definitely a case where "more is not better." Excessive drinking increases your risk of heart disease and stroke, as well as other health problems. The modest benefit that alcohol imparts on HDL may not warrant its other risks. Many people have health reasons that require complete avoidance of alcohol. Discuss alcohol use with your health-care provider.

> Unfortunately, there's no food you can eat that provides this "good" type of cholesterol. HDL is made in your body.

Elevated Homocysteine Levels

Homocysteine is an amino acid. Amino acids are the building blocks of proteins. Excessive amounts of homocysteine in the blood may be a potential risk factor for developing heart disease and stroke.

Studies have shown that certain vitamins can help to lower blood homocysteine levels. An adequate intake of folate, vitamin B6, and vitamin B12 can minimize your risk for heart disease.

- Foods high in folate include fruits and vegetables (especially leafy greens), legumes (dried beans), seaweed, avocado, yeast, wheat germ, and fortified cereals and grains. Strive for five servings per day from a combination of fruits and vegetables.

- Foods high in vitamin B6 include fortified cereals and grains, whole grains, brown rice, wheat germ, yeast, legumes, oats, bananas, potatoes, corn, avocados, sunflower seeds, fish, chicken, and lean pork.

- Foods high in vitamin B12 include all animal products such as meats, fish, poultry, eggs, milk, yogurt, and cheese. Strict vegetarians who avoid all animal products can ensure adequate B12 intake by including fortified grains and cereals in their diets or by taking vitamin B12 supplements.

Diabetes

Heart disease is the most common complication associated with diabetes. There are a number of contributing factors, and not all are well understood. Unfortunately, many people who get type 2 diabetes also inherit the genes that predispose them to hypertension, hyperlipidemia, and obesity. It's a "package deal" that has serious consequences. This type of genetic makeup greatly increases the risk of heart disease.

People with diabetes have some unique risk factors for heart disease. Insulin resistance is the hallmark of type 2 diabetes. The pancreas tries to compensate by making extra insulin. Insulin resistance and high levels of circulating insulin may damage the artery walls. Weight loss and exercise can combat insulin resistance and lower your risk for heart disease. Uncontrolled blood sugar can cause glycosylation,

> Your heart beats approximately 86,400 times per day. That's 31,536,000 heartbeats per year.

which can lead to heart disease and the other complications associated with diabetes. (Glycosylation is when the excess sugar in the blood permanently attaches to the blood vessels and body tissues.) Diabetes can also cause negative changes in coagulation (blood clotting), which increases the risk for heart attack and stroke. *Blood sugar control is crucial in preventing all diabetes complications, including heart disease.*

Obesity

Excess calories get converted to fat, which circulates in the bloodstream and gets stored in fat cells. The bottom line is: If you eat too many calories, you *will* gain weight. There are no two ways about it and it's not healthy. Obesity can lead to high triglycerides and high cholesterol, as well as low levels of the beneficial HDL cholesterol. Obesity can cause high blood pressure, insulin resistance, and type 2 diabetes. People who carry their extra pounds around the middle (apple-shaped) have a higher risk for heart disease than people who carry their excess weight in the buttocks and hips (pear shaped).

Fight obesity with a sensible weight management plan. Eat less fat, and reduce portion sizes to reduce calories. Include regular exercise. See chapter 9 for detailed weight control guidelines and chapter 10 for more information on exercise.

Physical Inactivity

Increasing your fitness level helps to reduce your risk for heart disease in several ways. First of all, the heart is a muscle and exercise can improve the fitness of the heart. Exercise is a key factor in reducing insulin resistance and therefore should be thought of as a foundation treatment for type 2 diabetes. Exercise is a key component of weight management, and it lowers the bad kinds of blood fats and helps to raise the HDL (good cholesterol). Exercise also helps to reduce blood pressure and improve circulation.

Many people who get type 2 diabetes also inherit the genes that predispose them to hypertension, hyperlipidemia, and obesity. It's a "package deal" that has serious consequences.

Exercise can be moderate and pleasurable. The main thing is that it has to be done on a regular basis. Get clearance from your health-care provider, start modestly, and work your way into regular physical activity. See chapter 10 for more information on exercise.

Tip: An aspirin a day may reduce your risk for heart attack. The usual dose is 81–325 milligrams of enteric-coated aspirin per day. Since aspirin therapy does carry some risks, ask your health-care provider if you should be on aspirin therapy.

Cholesterol and Fats in Food
Dietary Cholesterol

Cholesterol is produced in the liver (both in our livers and the livers of animals). It is then distributed throughout the body to carry on its specific functions. When you eat meat and other animal products, you eat the cholesterol that is contained in that food. Plants don't have cholesterol because they don't have livers to produce it. So, the next time you see an ad that says "Vegetable Oil—*No Cholesterol*," keep in mind that vegetable oil never had cholesterol in the first place. Cholesterol can only be made by animals, not plants. Hearing that, you may think, "Oh, great, now I have to be a vegetarian." Actually, meat can be a part of a healthful diet if you choose lean meats in reasonable portions. Cholesterol is found primarily in the red part of the meat, the flesh, not in the fat, so you can't cut it off. Some very lean meats have significant amounts of cholesterol. It's all about moderation and making healthful choices. Portion size will determine the amount of cholesterol that you eat. If your portion of meat is bigger than the size of the palm of your hand (twice a day), then you may be getting too much cholesterol. Eating too much dietary cholesterol can raise your blood cholesterol levels and contribute to clogged blood vessels and heart disease.

> People who carry their extra pounds around the middle (apple-shaped) have a higher risk for heart disease than people who carry their excess weight in the buttocks and hips (pear shaped).

Saturated Fat

Saturated fats are the kind that can raise your blood cholesterol. When you eat saturated fats, they're transported to your liver. The liver processes the fat and at the same time produces new cholesterol. The fats and cholesterol are then packaged together and sent into the bloodstream. You heard correctly: Eating saturated fat causes your liver to produce cholesterol! You can actually eat a food that boasts that it contains "no cholesterol," but if it contains saturated fat, you end up with more cholesterol in your blood anyway. Pretty sneaky. Luckily, saturated fats are easy to identify. They're either solid at room temperature, or they're the fats that come from animal products. Examples of solid fats are the white fat marbled in meat, chicken skin, cheese, butter, bacon fat, lard, coconut oil, palm oil, and palm kernel oil. Examples of saturated fats that are not solid but do come from animals are cream, whole milk, half & half, ice cream, and so on. *Limiting your intake of saturated fat is probably the most important dietary change that you can make to improve your blood cholesterol profile*. It will also help in your efforts to control your weight.

Hydrogenated Fat

Hydrogenation is the process of starting with liquid oil and adding hydrogen. This processing turns the liquid oil into a solid fat. Examples of hydrogenated fat include vegetable shortening and margarine. Both started as liquids and were turned into solids. A can of vegetable shortening may say "100% vegetable oil shortening" and "cholesterol free." Both statements may be true, but once you eat it, your liver kicks out its homemade cholesterol in the process. Solid fats, whether the saturated varieties mentioned previously or the hydrogenated varieties mentioned here, all hold the same potential danger for raising the blood cholesterol.

Trans-Fatty Acids

These types of fats are found primarily in the hydrogenated vegetable fats. Trans-fatty acids are considered bad because they can raise the LDL ("bad cholesterol") levels in the blood and lower the HDL ("good cholesterol") levels. As it turns out, butter and stick margarine are comparably bad for your blood cholesterol. The soft tub margarines are lower in both saturated fats and trans-fatty acids, which makes them the spread of choice. The softer the fat, the better for your blood cholesterol. Trans-fats are also commonly found in cookies, crackers, baked goods, and fried foods from restaurants.

> Eating saturated fat causes your liver to produce cholesterol! You can actually eat a food that boasts that it contains "no cholesterol," but if it contains saturated fat, then you end up with more cholesterol in your blood anyway.

Polyunsaturated Fat

Polyunsaturated fats do not raise the blood cholesterol. Vegetable oils are a primary source of polyunsaturated fat. Examples are soybean oil, safflower oil, corn oil, sunflower oil, sesame oil, and cottonseed oil. Although these oils do not raise your LDL ("bad cholesterol") levels, eating excess amounts can lower your HDL ("good cholesterol"). Use polyunsaturated vegetable oils in moderation.

Omega-3 Fatty Acids

Omega-3 fatty acids are a type of polyunsaturated fat that helps to lower blood cholesterol and blood fats (triglycerides). Omega-3 fats also help to thin the blood and prevent blood clots. Fish that come from cold, deep water are excellent sources of omega-3 fatty acid. Salmon, tuna, herring, sardines, and mackerel are among the richest sources. Eskimos traditionally ate a lot of fish and had very low rates of heart disease. So, eat fresh fish regularly! (Fish sticks, fried fish, and fast-food fish sandwiches are not your best choices because they have additional fat added.) Physicians may prescribe fish oil supplements to some individuals to combat very high blood triglyceride levels. The maximum dose is typically 2 grams per day.

If you don't like fish, vegetarian sources of omega-3 fatty acids are available. The best options include flaxseeds, flaxseed oil, walnuts, walnut oil, soybeans, soybean oil, canola oil, and evening primrose oil.

Monounsaturated Fat

Last, but certainly not least, comes monounsaturated fat. Monounsaturated fat does not negatively impact your blood cholesterol. The best sources are olive oil, canola oil, olives, avocados, peanuts, and peanut oil. These should be the types of fat you reach for most often. The diets of people living in Mediterranean countries are typically higher in monounsaturated fats and the prevalence of heart disease is lower than that in the United States. However, don't take that information as a license to overeat! Keep in mind that all fats have about the same number of calories. This means that one teaspoon of either butter, lard, or olive oil has approximately the same number of calories (45 calories, and 5 grams of fat per teaspoon). In other words, the effect on your *weight* is the same, no matter what type of fat you eat.

> Omega-3 fats also help to thin the blood and prevent blood clots. Fish that come from cold, deep water are excellent sources of omega-3 fatty acid.

Recommendations for Dietary Cholesterol Intake

New guidelines from the National Cholesterol Education Program say that you should limit your intake of dietary cholesterol to no more than 200 milligrams per day. Use table 11.5 to see how your cholesterol intake adds up. Grams of total fat and saturated fat are also listed.

You may be surprised to see how much cholesterol is in liver. Remember that *the liver is the organ that makes cholesterol*. When you eat liver, you're eating the manufacturing and packaging plant that produces cholesterol. Liver is chock-full of vitamins and minerals, but you may wish to weigh the pros and cons before eating it frequently.

Table 11.5   Cholesterol and Fat Content for Select Foods

(Values rounded to the nearest whole number)

Food	Portion	Cholesterol (mg)	Total Fat (g)	Saturated Fat (g)
Dairy Products				
Milk (nonfat)	1 cup	4	0	0
Milk (lowfat)	1 cup	10	3	2
Milk (whole)	1 cup	33	8	5
Yogurt (nonfat)	1 cup	10	0	0
Yogurt (whole)	1 cup	29	7	5
Cheddar cheese	1 oz.	30	9	6
Cottage cheese (lowfat)	1 cup	10	2	2
Fats				
Butter	1 tsp.	11	4	3
Margarine	1 tsp.	0	4	1
Vegetable oils	1 tsp.	0	5	1–2
Meats and Protein Foods				
Tofu	½ cup	0	11	2
Pinto beans	½ cup	0	1	0
Egg	1	212	5	2
Halibut	3½ oz.	41	3	–
Salmon	3½ oz.	63	12	2
Oysters	3½ oz.	55	2	1
Crab	3½ oz.	52	1	–
Lobster	3½ oz.	71	1	–
Tuna (in water)	3½ oz.	30	1	–
Shrimp	3½ oz.	194	1	–
Squid	3½ oz.	231	1	–
Beef (ground, lean)	3½ oz.	78	18	7
Beef (short ribs)	3½ oz.	94	42	18
Beef (sirloin)	3½ oz.	89	12	5
Beef Liver	3½ oz.	389	5	2
Veal (top round)	3½ oz.	135	5	2
Lamb (foreshank)	3½ oz.	106	14	6
Ham	3½ oz.	53	6	2
Pork (tenderloin)	3½ oz.	79	6	2
Pork (chop)	3½ oz.	85	25	10
Chicken Liver	3½ oz.	631	6	2
Chicken (white, no skin)	3½ oz.	85	5	1

Fruits, vegetables, grains, and all other plant foods do not have any cholesterol at all!

Some surprise contenders in the high cholesterol arena are shrimp and squid, weighing in at 194 and 231 mg, respectively. Liver, shrimp, and squid are all lowfat meats, yet they're high in cholesterol. Notice that chicken has similar amounts of cholesterol to other types of meat. Chicken is low in fat, but portion control is important when trying to stay within the budget for dietary cholesterol. Besides watching cholesterol intake, continue to limit the saturated fats found in meats. Do this by buying lean meats. The high cholesterol content in eggs is from the yolks, not the whites. Egg whites are low in both fat and cholesterol and high in protein.

The real key is making dietary substitutions that are lower in both cholesterol and saturated fat. Finding an alternate that tastes good and is good for you is the best solution. The good news is that supermarkets are full of more healthful choices. Many people find that giving up a favorite food completely just doesn't work in the long run. If you can't find an acceptable substitution, try cutting back on the regular variety by eating smaller portions or choosing it less often.

> Remember that the liver is the organ that makes cholesterol. When you eat liver, you're eating the manufacturing and packaging plant that produces cholesterol.

See chapter 21, "Eat Well, Be Well," for practical tips on cutting fat and cholesterol. Shopping, cooking, and dining strategies are covered.

Soluble Fiber

A diet rich in soluble fiber has been shown to help decrease blood cholesterol values. Here's how it works. When you eat foods that contain soluble fiber, the fiber forms a gel as it moves through the intestines. Bile, a digestive juice, gets trapped in the gelled soluble fiber. Bile is normally reabsorbed in the intestine and reused over and over again, but when it gets trapped in the soluble fiber, it gets eliminated with the stool. Once the bile is eliminated, the body must make more bile. It makes new bile by taking cholesterol out of the blood, and converting it to bile in the liver. The net effect is that the blood cholesterol ends up being lowered. Foods high in soluble fiber include oat bran, oatmeal, beans, peas, lentils, rice bran, barley, carrots, broccoli, sweet potatoes, citrus fruits, papayas, strawberries, and apples. Psyllium fiber supplements also do the trick. Some medications, known as bile acid sequesterants, are prescribed to do this same thing. See chapter 18 for more information on fiber.

Summary of Heart-Healthy Dietary Tips

Are you feeling confused about what to eat? Here are a few points that can help to keep your heart healthy:

- Cut down on saturated fats (animal fats and solid fats).
- Limit high-cholesterol foods to occasional use.
- Use leaner selections of meat.
- Keep your portion of meat no larger than the palm of your hand (twice a day).
- Use nonfat or lowfat dairy products.
- Limit added fats.
- Use lowfat cooking methods.
- Limit fried foods.
- Limit egg yolks to 3–4 per week.
- Use egg whites or cholesterol-free egg substitutes.
- Eat a diet rich in fruits, vegetables, beans, and oats.
- Include more fresh fish in your diet.

CHAPTER 12

The Pressure's On:
Controlling Hypertension

⟡

IN THIS CHAPTER

- Understanding blood pressure
- What do the numbers mean?
- Who gets high blood pressure?
- What are the risk factors?
- Treating high blood pressure

If you have high blood pressure, you aren't alone. Nearly one out of
every four adults in the United States has high blood pressure, and
many don't even know it. You don't have to be stressed out, high-strung,
or overworked to have high blood pressure. It can happen to anyone.
Although doctors don't always know exactly what causes high blood
pressure, many things can be done to treat it.

High blood pressure, also called hypertension, is a silent disease.
It often exists without any symptoms. You may ask, If it doesn't hurt,
why fix it? Elevated blood pressure is dangerous. High blood pressure causes the heart to work harder. Eventually, the heart may become
enlarged. The heart muscle can become over-stretched and weak-
ened and that can lead to heart failure. High blood pressure can also
damage arteries and contribute to atherosclerosis (hardening of the

173

arteries) and coronary heart disease. Not only does high blood pressure increase your risk of heart disease, it can also lead to kidney disease, eye disease, and stroke. Uncontrolled hypertension greatly increases the risks of getting diabetes-related complications. Controlling blood pressure is every bit as important as controlling blood sugar.

You don't have to be stressed out, high-strung, or overworked to have high blood pressure. It can happen to anyone.

People with type 2 diabetes are twice as likely to have high blood pressure. In fact, a cluster of health problems tends to occur together. This phenomenon is known as syndrome X. The package deal includes diabetes (or insulin resistance), high levels of the bad type of cholesterol (LDL), low levels of the good type of cholesterol (HDL), high triglycerides (blood fats), obesity, high blood pressure, and atherosclerosis (hardening of the arteries). To have all of these problems can be overwhelming. Just take it one step at a time. The good news is that all of these things are treatable. Better news yet—treating one problem may lead to improvements in other areas. For example, losing weight helps improve the diabetes and, at the same time, also helps to lower the cholesterol and the blood pressure.

Understanding Blood Pressure

When the heart beats, it pumps blood into the arteries (blood vessels). As blood is forced into the arteries, the artery walls resist and pressure is created within the arteries. This pressure allows the blood to flow throughout the body. The pressure is the highest when the heart contracts, and the pressure falls when the heart relaxes between beats.

Having your blood pressure checked is simple and painless. A rubber cuff is placed around the upper arm and the cuff is inflated to compress the blood flow in the arm (see figure 12.1). Then the cuff pressure is released and the blood starts to flow freely again. The healthcare provider listens to the sound of the blood flow while looking at the pressure gauge. It's that easy. If you haven't had your blood pressure checked, be sure to do so soon.

Figure 12.1—Blood Pressure Meter

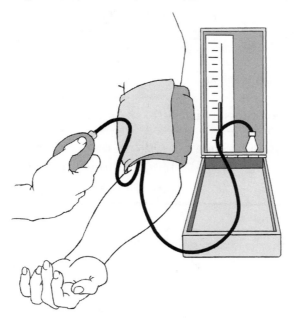

What Do the Numbers Mean?

Blood pressure values are expressed as one number over another number—for example, 120/80. (Blood pressure is measured in millimeters of mercury, which is abbreviated mmHg.)

- *Systolic:* The top number is the systolic pressure and represents the peak pressure during the heart's contraction.

- *Diastolic:* The bottom number is the diastolic pressure and represents the pressure when the heart is resting between contractions.

Blood pressure can change throughout the day in relation to your activity level. It varies, depending on whether you're lying down, sitting, or standing. Stress and anxiety can also affect your readings.

When you compare your blood pressure number to table 12.1, keep in mind that your top number (systolic blood pressure) may fall into one category, and your bottom number (diastolic blood pressure) may fall into another category. Blood pressure is still considered high if *either* the

**Table 12.1   Blood Pressure Values for Adults
(Values Expressed in mmHg)**

Optimal blood pressure is less than 120/80.
Normal blood pressure is less than 130/85.
High-normal blood pressure is 130/85 through 139/89.
High blood pressure: Stage 1: 140/90 through 159/99 Stage 2: 160/100 through 179/109 Stage 3: 180/110 or higher

systolic number *or* the diastolic number is elevated. For example, a blood pressure reading of 166/88 would be classified as stage 2 hypertension even though only the systolic number falls in the stage 2 category.

Tip: If you have diabetes, it's recommended that you achieve a blood pressure target of less than 130/80. The risk for problems associated with hypertension is lowest when the blood pressure is less than 120/80.

Who Gets High Blood Pressure?

One out of every four American adults has high blood pressure. If you are African American, make that one out of every three people. High blood pressure tends to run in families. It strikes more often in people over 35 years old, and by age 65, more than half of us will have high blood pressure. Women are especially susceptible after menopause. Birth control pills may cause high blood pressure in some women. Although more common in adults, hypertension can still affect young adults and even children.

What Are the Risk Factors?

The confirmed risk factors for hypertension include:

- Being overweight
- Not exercising enough

- Drinking too much alcohol
- Eating too much salt

Other Risk Factors for Developing Hypertension: Fact or Fiction?

- *Does stress cause high blood pressure?*
  Blood pressure can go up temporarily during a stressful event. Emotional stress does not cause persistently high blood pressure. Nevertheless, stress-reduction techniques can't hurt.

- *Does caffeine cause high blood pressure?*
  If you drink enough caffeine, the blood pressure may go up temporarily. Most coffee drinkers get accustomed to their caffeine intake, and the blood pressure loses interest in responding.

- *Does smoking cause high blood pressure?*
  Blood pressure goes up every time you light up. Smoking is a major risk factor in developing heart disease and other diseases. If you smoke, ask your doctor to refer you to a smoking cessation program.

Treating High Blood Pressure

Healthful living can mean better blood pressure. The lifestyle strategies to prevent and treat high blood pressure are straightforward: Watch your weight, stay active, limit alcohol, and eat right. These same strategies are important in caring for your diabetes and your heart, as well as your general health.

Achieve and Maintain a Reasonable Weight

Being overweight increases the likelihood of having high blood pressure by as much as sixfold. Carrying the extra weight around your middle (apple-shaped) holds more risks than carrying your weight around your hips (pear-shaped). If you're overweight, it's important to lose weight.

Even losing a modest amount of weight can greatly improve blood pressure values. Think in small steps. Aim for losing 5 pounds, and then, when you achieve that, aim for 5 more pounds. Continue making small steps until you reach a reasonable weight.

Ten Things You Can Do to Lose Weight

1.   Limit fried foods.
2.   Choose leaner cuts of meat.
3.   Take the skin off chicken and turkey.
4.   Choose nonfat or lowfat dairy products.
5.   Read food labels. Choose items with 3 grams of fat or less.
6.   Look for nonfat, fat-free, lowfat, and reduced-fat products.
7.   Limit added fats such as butter, margarine, mayo, and oils.
8.   Use lowfat cooking methods: bake, broil, boil, steam, poach, and grill.
9.   Steer clear of fast-food restaurants.
10. Include regular exercise.

See chapter 9 for more weight management strategies.

Keep Active

Exercise, if done regularly, has wonderful benefits. Exercise reduces blood pressure, reduces the risk of heart disease, improves blood sugar control, and is important in achieving and maintaining a reasonable weight.

Moderate exercise such as brisk walking is recommended, but you can choose any aerobic activity that you enjoy. Other choices might include dancing, bicycling, swimming, or aerobics classes or videos.

The general recommendation is to strive for 30 minutes of exercise per day. That can be all at once, or divided into two or three sessions throughout the day. Try to exercise on most days of the week.

Caution: Be sure to discuss your intention to exercise with your health-care provider to see if any restrictions or safety precautions apply to you. If you have diabetic eye disease, you must be careful not to do exercises that cause you to strain, such as heavy weight lifting. Intense straining can cause an acute rise in blood pressure that can damage the small blood vessels in the eyes.

> People with type 2 diabetes are twice as likely to have high blood pressure.

An exercise stress test is recommended for anyone over 35 years old; anyone who has had diabetes for 10 years; anyone with preexisting diabetes complications; or anyone with risk factors for heart disease.

Ten Ways to Add Activity to Your Day

1. Do errands by foot, or by bicycle, when reasonable to do so.
2. Take the stairs.
3. Walk the dog.
4. Buy a stationary bike, treadmill, or other exercise equipment for use at home.
5. Buy an exercise video, and use it regularly!
6. Finish your meal with a walk instead of dessert!
7. Join an exercise class.
8. Enlist an exercise buddy who will join you for regularly scheduled exercise.
9. Tune in to an exercise program on TV, and participate.
10. Join a gym.

See chapter 10 for more information on exercise.

Limit Alcohol

If you drink, do so in moderation. Excessive amounts of alcohol pose many health risks. Too much alcohol can increase your risk for stroke, hypertension, heart disease, liver disease, diseases of the pancreas, accidents, and the list goes on.

One way to take care of your blood pressure is to make sure you don't exceed one to two drinks per day. A maximum of one drink is recommended if you are a woman or if you have a small body size. A maximum of two drinks is recommended if you are a man or if you have a larger body size.

Tip: One drink is considered 12 ounces of beer, 5 ounces of wine, or 1½ ounces of 80 proof hard liquor.

Caution: Check with your health-care provider to find out if it's okay for you to include a limited amount of alcohol in your diet. Certain health problems and medications require a complete avoidance of alcohol.

Ten Ways to Curb Your Alcohol Intake

1. Use a shot glass to measure your distilled spirits.
2. Use a measuring cup to pour a 5-ounce glass of wine.
3. Order singles instead of doubles.
4. Choose non-alcoholic beer. (Some great ones are on the market.)
5. Make a virgin Bloody Mary with low-sodium tomato juice.
6. Have a diet tonic with lime. Skip the gin.
7. Try the "every other" system—one non-alcoholic beverage before and between your alcoholic beverage choices.
8. Bring non-alcoholic beverages to parties to make sure you have options.
9. Choose non-alcoholic diet drinks such as diet soda, mineral water, or iced tea.
10. Avoid situations and places that make it difficult to stick to your limit.

See chapter 19 for more alcohol advice.

Limit Salt

Although the terms *salt* and *sodium* are used interchangeably, they aren't exactly the same thing. Salt is made from sodium and chloride. It's 40 percent sodium and 60 percent chloride by weight. Excessive intake of sodium is linked to elevation in blood pressure. Sodium occurs naturally in many foods, but most of our sodium intake comes from added salt.

The average American eats up to 6,000 milligrams of sodium per day. It's estimated that about 75 percent of that sodium comes from packaged and processed foods. In addition to flavoring foods, salt is a preservative and is added to processed foods to improve shelf life.

High blood pressure tends to run in families. It strikes more often in people over 35 years old, and by age 65, more than half of us will have high blood pressure.

Convenience foods, as the name implies, are convenient, but they also tend to be high in sodium. If making dinner involves adding hot water, stirring, and waiting 5 minutes, then you'd better take a second look at that food label. Chances are you're in for a high-sodium meal. The same holds true if you pick up your meal at a drive-through window. Quick meals don't have to be high in sodium, but to limit sodium you do have to rethink your choices.

As a part of a healthful diet, the recommended limit for sodium intake is 2,400 milligrams per day. Individuals vary in their sensitivity to salt. Lowering dietary sodium intake will benefit some people's blood pressure more than others. Compared to the general population, people with diabetes do tend to have a better response to a low-sodium diet.

Start by shopping for foods low in sodium. Try to use more unprocessed, fresh foods. When buying packaged foods, read the labels for the sodium content.

- Sodium-free is less than 5 mg per serving.
- Very low sodium is less than 35 mg per serving.
- Low sodium is less than 140 mg per serving.

By the way, one teaspoon of salt has more than 2,300 mg of sodium! So, try not to add salt. Use other seasonings to bring out the flavor in foods.

Ten Ways to Cut Down on Salt

1. Get rid of your salt shaker!
2. Season with fresh or dried herbs.
3. Try adding lemon, garlic, ginger, onions, or flavored vinegar.
4. Look for low sodium, reduced sodium, or "no salt added" products.
5. Don't add salt to the cooking water for rice, pasta, or cooked cereals.
6. Make homemade soups, or buy low-sodium canned soups.
7. Rinse canned foods that have been processed with added salt.
8. Buy salt-free seasoning shakers.
9. Limit salted convenience foods like instant rice, pasta, and potato dishes.
10. Steer clear of fast-food restaurants.

See chapter 21 for more low sodium strategies.

Other Dietary Tips to Improve Blood Pressure

High-Potassium Diet

> Excessive intake of sodium is linked to elevation in blood pressure.

A diet high in potassium may help reduce the risk of high blood pressure. As of October 2000 the FDA (U.S. Food and Drug Administration) allows food labels to claim that foods high in potassium and low in sodium may reduce the risk of high blood pressure and stroke. The label claim can only be used on foods that have at least 350 mg of potassium and no more than 140 mg of sodium.

Which Foods Are Naturally High in Potassium?

Apricots, avocados, bananas, cantaloupe, kiwi, mangos, oranges, strawberries, artichokes, tomatoes, potatoes, sweet potatoes, legumes (peas, lentils, and beans), parsnips, winter squashes, milk, yogurt, meat, poultry, and fish are all good sources of potassium.

Caution: Certain blood pressure medications can alter blood levels of potassium (causing you to either retain too much potassium or lose too much potassium). If you take blood pressure medications, ask your health-care provider if you need to be concerned about your dietary potassium intake.

> If making dinner involves adding hot water, stirring, and waiting 5 minutes, then you'd better take a second look at that food label. Chances are you're in for a high-sodium meal.

People with kidney disease are often prescribed low-potassium diets and must limit high-potassium foods.

Tip: Salt substitutes are often made from potassium chloride. If you have medical reasons to limit potassium intake, then you shouldn't use potassium chloride salt substitutes.

Adequate Calcium Intake

Studies have shown that diets low in calcium are often associated with an increased incidence of hypertension. Other studies fail to show a clear-cut relationship between calcium and blood pressure. At this point, it seems safe to say that including calcium-rich foods is prudent, but calcium supplementation is not a proven therapy for lowering blood pressure.

Which Foods Are Naturally High in Calcium?

Milk, yogurt, and cheese are the richest sources of calcium. You can also buy calcium-fortified tofu and soy milk. Legumes (dried beans, split peas, and lentils), broccoli, and cooked greens such as kale, spinach, and mustard greens offer some calcium.

Adequate Magnesium Intake

Inadequate magnesium intake may contribute to high blood pressure, though studies are not conclusive enough to suggest magnesium supplementation. Including dietary sources of magnesium-rich foods may be beneficial.

> Studies have shown that diets low in calcium are often associated with an increased incidence of hypertension. Other studies fail to show a clear-cut relationship between calcium and blood pressure.

Which Foods Are Naturally High in Magnesium?

Leafy green vegetables, legumes (dried beans, split peas, and lentils), whole grains, and nuts and seeds.

Fish Oils

Omega-3 fatty acid is a type of fat that may help to reduce high blood pressure. Include fresh fish regularly to cash in on this benefit.

Which Types of Fish Are Rich in Omega-3 Fatty Acids?

Fish that come from cold, deep water are an excellent source of omega-3 fatty acid. Salmon, tuna, herring, sardines, and mackerel are among the richest sources.

Treating High Blood Pressure with Medication

Many types of medications can be used to lower the blood pressure. If lifestyle modifications haven't corrected your blood pressure, it's time to ask your doctor about blood pressure–lowering medications. Medications are often used in combination, so don't be discouraged if you need to take more than one type of pill to successfully lower your blood pressure. In the meantime, keep up the healthful lifestyle: watch your weight, exercise regularly, and limit alcohol and sodium.

Take your medications as prescribed. Don't stop taking your medication when your blood pressure falls into target range. Achieving normal blood pressure numbers on medication doesn't mean that it's time to stop taking the pills; it means the pills are working! If you're having undesirable side effects from your blood pressure medications, report your concerns to your health-care provider. You may tolerate a different type of medication better.

Summary

- Have your blood pressure checked regularly.

- Lose weight if you're overweight.

- Increase your level of activity. Exercise regularly. Strive for at least 30 minutes per day.

- Limit alcohol to no more than one to two drinks per day. Choose non-alcoholic beverages.

- Eat less salt. Choose unsalted foods and products that claim to be low in sodium.

- Ensure an adequate intake of dietary potassium, calcium, and magnesium.

- Take blood pressure medications as directed by your health-care provider.

- Don't smoke.

CHAPTER 13

Kids Get Type 2, Too

❧

IN THIS CHAPTER

- High-fat diets and sedentary lifestyles contribute to childhood obesity
- Risk factors for developing type 2 diabetes in childhood
- Screening for diabetes in children
- Treatment goals for children with diabetes
- Treatment strategies
- Diabetes in the school setting
- Preventing type 2 diabetes in children
- Book list

High-Fat Diets and Sedentary Lifestyles Contribute to Childhood Obesity

Type 2 diabetes was once considered an adult-only disease. Not anymore. Every year the number of cases of type 2 diabetes in children and adolescents increases. Why? Because kids are getting heavier and are exercising less.

To illustrate, I'd like to tell you about a 15-year-old Hispanic girl who recently visited our clinic, accompanied by her parents. She was

5'3" and weighed 170 pounds. She had just been diagnosed with type 2 diabetes. A high-fat diet contributed to her obesity. As in many high schools, her school lunch choices included pizza, cheeseburgers, corn dogs, french fries, and other high-fat foods. She usually drank a large soft drink with lunch and opted for cookies or a candy bar for dessert. After school, she snacked while doing her homework. Typical snack foods included chips, ice cream, or cookies and more soft drinks. Her family enjoyed traditional Mexican foods. On the plus side, she regularly ate fruits and vegetables, but on the minus side, many of the family's entrees were high in fat, fried, or made with high-fat cheeses. Her evenings were often spent watching television. She had several close friends, but otherwise kept to herself. She was teased at school for being overweight and often felt depressed. She was self-conscious of her weight and felt awkward participating in gym class.

> The rate of obesity among American children has more than doubled in the last 25 years. One out of every four children is overweight or obese.

The treatment plan for this 15-year-old girl included educating her and her parents on healthful food choices. She agreed to pack her own lunch three days a week and buy school lunch only two days a week. She agreed to switch to diet sodas. We explored more healthful snack options, including baked chips, fresh fruit, raw vegetables with fat-free dips, rice cakes, and microwave light popcorn. She was interested in trying nonfat, no-sugar-added puddings, yogurts, and fudge pops. Instead of eliminating the traditional foods that she enjoyed, we discussed lowfat cooking methods and recipe modification tips to reduce fat content and calories. Since she was very sedentary, we agreed she'd start walking 20 minutes, at least three days per week. Eventually, the goal would be 30 minutes of activity, five days per week. Her mother said that she would go on the walks, too. Both parents agreed to purchase more healthful snacks and prepare lower-fat meals. The family members also met with the nurse to learn how to monitor the blood sugar at home. They met with the social worker, who helped them explore the feelings surrounding this new diagnosis. They also met with the pediatric endocrinologist, who did a full physical exam, ordered more lab tests, and decided to monitor the effects of dietary changes and exercise before starting any medications. The family would return in four weeks to continue their education and evaluate the child's progress.

Her story isn't uncommon. The rate of obesity among American children has more than doubled in the last 25 years. One out of every four children is overweight or obese. Kids are eating too many foods that are low in fiber and high in fat or sugar. Fast-food chains and manufacturers of snack foods target their advertisements to children. High-fat fast foods, convenience foods, and snack foods are often poor choices nutritionally, and to make matters worse, they now come in giant and super sizes! A "small" soda has grown to 16 ounces! The school lunch program has taken a nose-dive in many districts. Fewer schools offer healthful, lowfat entrees. More schools contract out to fast-food vendors to supply menu items. Kids drink less milk and more soft drinks with their school lunches. Schools are cutting physical education classes as their budgets tighten. Kids spend more time plugged into television, computers, and electronic games and less time engaged in physical activity. A child who watches four or more hours of television per day is 2.5 times more likely to be obese than a child who watches one hour or less of television per day.

> As the incidence of obesity rises, the incidence of obesity-related diseases rises. Type 2 diabetes, high blood pressure, and high cholesterol are all associated with obesity and threaten potential long-term complications.

Things won't change until we all make some noise. Limit television time. Ask the schools to reinstate physical education classes and after-school sports. Petition your schools to provide healthful menus. Write to the fast-food chains and request more healthful menu items. How hard can it be to come up with a lower-fat kid's meal that includes some fresh fruit or vegetables?

Obesity is becoming an epidemic. As the incidence of obesity rises, the incidence of obesity-related diseases rises. Type 2 diabetes, high blood pressure, and high cholesterol are all associated with obesity and threaten potential long-term complications. The duration of diabetes is a strong predictor of risk for developing complications. How much more likely is someone to develop complications if that person is diagnosed with type 2 diabetes at age 15 instead of age 45? No one knows for sure, but giving type 2 diabetes a 30-year head start can't help. Fortunately, we have good studies showing that complications are preventable. We know that controlling the blood sugar, the blood pressure, and the blood cholesterol is critical in preventing complications. Appropriate education, treatment, and control must start immediately.

> Excess body fat leads to insulin resistance. Insulin resistance means that the body's own insulin doesn't work properly at controlling the blood sugar.

Risk Factors for Developing Type 2 Diabetes in Childhood

Type 2 Diabetes Runs in Families

- 45–80 percent of children who develop type 2 diabetes have a parent with type 2 diabetes.
- 75–100 percent of children who develop type 2 diabetes have a relative with type 2 diabetes.

Certain Racial Groups Are at Higher Risk for Developing Type 2 Diabetes

- Native American
- African American
- Hispanic American

- Asian American
- Pacific Islander

Obesity Greatly Increases the Risk of Developing Type 2 Diabetes

Excess body fat leads to insulin resistance. Insulin resistance means that the body's own insulin doesn't work properly at controlling the blood sugar. High-fat diets and sedentary lifestyles increase the risk of obesity, which in turn increases the risk of developing type 2 diabetes.

Puberty

Children who develop type 2 diabetes usually do so after age 10 or when puberty kicks in. The changing hormone levels associated with puberty cause increased insulin resistance.

Several conditions are associated with insulin resistance. The presence of one of the following conditions increases the likelihood of getting type 2 diabetes.

- *Acanthosis nigricans* is present in about 90 percent of children who have type 2 diabetes. Acanthosis nigricans is a condition of dark, thickened, or shiny patches on the skin. It may look like a band of darkened skin across the back of the neck, under the armpits, or between the fingers or toes.

- *Polycystic ovary syndrome (PCOS):* PCOS is a condition that results in excess production of specific types of hormones called androgens. Females with PCOS tend to be overweight and insulin-resistant.

- *High blood pressure:* Children who are overweight tend to have higher blood pressure than lean children do. High blood pressure may be inherited. High blood pressure is more common in African Americans than in any other group. It's recommended that all children have their blood pressure checked at least annually.

- *Blood fat disorders:* Individuals with diabetes often have abnormalities in cholesterol and blood fats. Disorders include elevated levels of the bad kinds of cholesterol (LDL cholesterol and VLDL cholesterol), elevated blood fats (triglycerides), or reduced levels of the good kind of cholesterol (HDL cholesterol).

Screening for Diabetes in Children

Any child who exhibits symptoms of diabetes, or any child who is at risk for developing type 2 diabetes, should be screened. The problem with type 2 diabetes is that it can go unnoticed for years. Many children are walking around undiagnosed. Don't assume that your child will have symptoms. And don't wait for your child's pediatrician to bring up the subject. Be proactive, and ask for the test.

> The problem with type 2 diabetes is that it can go unnoticed for years. Many children are walking around undiagnosed.

Tip: Children who are at risk for developing diabetes should be screened every two years.

Who's at Risk and Should Be Screened?

All children who are overweight or over 10 years old should be screened every two years if they have any two of the following risk factors:

- Has a family history of type 2 diabetes
- Is a member of a high-risk ethnic group
- Has high blood pressure
- Has high cholesterol or high triglycerides
- Has polycystic ovary syndrome (PCOS)
- Has acanthosis nigricans

The Screening Test

A blood test is used to diagnose diabetes. The blood is drawn first thing in the morning after a child has gone at least 8 hours without eating or drinking anything (except water). If the blood sugar is 126 mg/dl (milligrams per deciliter) or higher, the diagnosis of diabetes is made. If the blood sugar is checked after eating, or any other nonfasting time, a reading of 200 mg/dl or greater indicates diabetes. Further blood tests can be done to distinguish type 1 diabetes from type 2 diabetes.

Responsibility for diabetes care should be shared between the child and caretakers. Instead of considering it "the child's diabetes," consider it "the family's diabetes."

Caution: Impaired glucose tolerance (IGT) is when the blood glucose readings are higher than normal but not yet high enough to be called type 2 diabetes. IGT often leads to type 2 diabetes in the future. IGT is defined as a fasting blood glucose value of 110–125 mg/dl, or a post-meal blood glucose value of 140–199 mg/dl.

Fasting blood sugar of 126 mg/dl or higher indicates diabetes.

Nonfasting blood sugar of 200 mg/dl or higher indicates diabetes.

Sorting Out the Type of Diabetes

Children can get two main types of diabetes: type 1 diabetes (which used to be called juvenile-onset diabetes) and type 2 diabetes (which used to be called adult-onset diabetes). Here are the key characteristics:

Type 1 Diabetes

- Majority of individuals are normal weight.
- Highest incidence is in individuals with Scandinavian ancestry.
- Usually develops in childhood (but can also develop in adults).
- Onset is associated with significant weight loss, thirst, and frequent urination.

- Must take insulin injections for life.
- Lack of insulin can lead to ketone production, which if left untreated leads to nausea, vomiting, and ketoacidosis (a life-threatening condition where acids build up in the blood).

Type 2 Diabetes

- Majority of individuals are overweight.
- Highest incidence is with African Americans, Hispanic Americans, Native Americans, Asian Americans, or Pacific Islanders.
- Usually develops in adults (but can also develop in childhood).
- Onset may, or may not, have symptoms such as thirst and frequent urination.
- May be controlled by diet modifications and exercise in some individuals.
- May require pills or insulin for effective control in other individuals.
- Usually not prone to forming ketones (acids in the blood).

Treatment Goals for Children with Diabetes

- Achieve blood sugar levels as close to normal as possible.
- Hemoglobin A1c levels as close to normal as possible. (This test indicates average blood sugar control over the past 2–3 months.)
- Appropriate growth without excessive weight gain.
- Prevention of complications.
- Treatment of associated disorders.
- Quality of life and psychosocial well-being.

Treatment Strategies

Most of the basic treatment principles discussed in chapter 2 apply to adults as well as to children with type 2 diabetes. The following additional information on treating diabetes pertains specifically to children and adolescents and can be reviewed in addition to the information provided in chapter 2.

Parenting Pointers

Parenting a child with diabetes takes knowledge, skill, patience, trust, finesse, courage, hope, support, discipline, and a great deal of responsibility. No one will tell you it's easy. At first, the brunt of the responsibility for diabetes care falls on the parents. As children get older, they can begin to take on age-appropriate diabetes self-management tasks. The transfer of responsibility from parent to child is a tricky dance. Despite the fact that some children are quite capable of performing diabetes-related tasks themselves, parents should not relinquish their support and supervision. It's crucial that the child isn't overly burdened too soon. Kids can get burned out. They don't get a vacation from diabetes. Responsibility for diabetes care should be shared between the child and caretakers. Instead of considering it "the child's diabetes," consider it "the family's diabetes."

> I don't like to use the word *diet* when describing meal planning. Diet sounds temporary and it sounds negative.

Adolescence is a tricky time, when parents must supervise and support yet give up some of the control. Teens tend to be risk-takers and feel as if they're indestructible. They want to fit in. They don't want to be different and may not want their friends to know they have diabetes. Caregivers must convey the importance of diabetes self-management without using scare tactics. Don't threaten a child with diabetes complications. Fear isn't a good motivator and can actually leave the child feeling, "Why bother?" Children need praise and reinforcement. Use positive motivators such as allowing the child to earn a privilege for performing diabetes tasks. Let kids know that blood sugar control improves the ability to concentrate and do well in school. Well-controlled blood sugar also reduces fatigue and allows peak athletic performance. One thing has become evident to me; the kids who receive the most support and supervision tend to have the best blood sugar control.

Education and Medical Follow-Up

Diabetes management has many facets. Seek out health-care providers who specialize in diabetes. If at all possible, enlist the help of a health-care *team*, including, but not limited to, a pediatric endocrinologist, a nurse educator, a registered dietitian, and a counselor or social worker. Look for health-care providers who specialize in pediatrics. (Children are not just small adults.)

Have regular follow-ups. A common schedule is a medical follow-up at least every three to four months. (Your health-care team may suggest more, or less, frequent visits.) Children and adolescents have changing needs. Medical management has to keep up with blood sugar fluctuations caused by growth and development, hormonal changes, schedule changes, and variations in exercise and activity.

Hemoglobin A1c levels should be checked every three months to monitor blood sugar control. (This is in *addition to*, not *instead of*, home blood sugar monitoring. See chapter 2 for more information on blood sugar monitoring.)

> Don't threaten a child with diabetes complications. Fear isn't a good motivator and can actually leave the child feeling, "Why bother?"

It's important for *both* parents to know how to care for their child's diabetes. Whenever possible, both parents should come to the child's medical visits. Grandparents, day-care providers, teachers, and baby-sitters also must know the nuts and bolts of diabetes care, in order to provide consistent and safe care for the child with diabetes.

Education is an ongoing process. Diabetes necessitates many skills and self-management strategies, often requiring significant behavior change. Behavior change is a gradual process and is best approached in a step-wise fashion.

Adolescents must be counseled on the risks of smoking. Besides its many health risks, smoking greatly increases the chances of developing diabetic complications. Adolescents must also be counseled on the risks of alcohol. In addition to the obvious dangers, alcohol poses special hazards for individuals who inject insulin or take certain types of diabetes medications. See chapter 19 for more information on alcohol.

Adolescent girls must be educated regarding unplanned pregnancy. Uncontrolled maternal blood sugar levels in early pregnancy can lead to fetal malformations and birth defects. (For more information on pregnancy and diabetes, see chapter 14.)

Routine eye exams and kidney function tests must be performed. High blood pressure, high cholesterol, and depression should be treated aggressively.

Meal Planning

I don't like to use the word *diet* when describing meal planning. Diet sounds temporary and it sounds negative. The nutritional management of diabetes involves establishing healthful eating behaviors that should last a lifetime. It's important for parents to demonstrate healthful eating behaviors. Kids learn many eating habits from their parents.

A review of the typical child's diet in our country reveals a sad picture indeed. Most kids eat less fruits and vegetables and more fat than is recommended. Fast foods and convenience foods are contributing to the obesity crisis in our youth. Kids are skipping important meals like breakfast and lunch and filling up on high-sugar and high-fat snack foods.

Here are a few suggestions to improve childhood nutrition:

- Don't skip meals. Eat three meals per day (plus snacks if desired).

- Choose healthful, lowfat snacks.

- Strive for five! Choose at least five servings per day from a combination of fruits and vegetables.

- Choose lean meats and lowfat dairy products.

- Limit added fats and fried foods.

- Try to use foods higher in fiber and water content.

- Eat fewer fast-food meals. Consider fast food *fat food*.

- Discourage eating out of boredom or for emotional reasons.

- Limit eating in front of the television.

- Choose diet soft drinks instead of regular sodas and sugary beverages.

- Don't force kids to clean their plates! Provide healthful menu selections and let kids choose from those selections and choose how much they want to eat. Children need to learn to quit eating when they're full, by following their appetite cues.

> A review of the typical child's diet in our country reveals a sad picture indeed. Most kids eat less fruits and vegetables and more fat than is recommended.

Kids with diabetes are still kids! It's important to incorporate favorite foods in reasonable amounts, even if those foods aren't the most healthful choices. It's all about moderation. If a child has a well-balanced, healthful diet most of the time, that's what counts. There's room to fit a candy bar or a couple of cookies into the meal plan. Besides, if you don't negotiate the inclusion of some favored items, those items tend to get eaten anyway. The kids just don't tell you. It's better to fit the item in at a designated snack time or mealtime. Treats can be traded for the usual carbohydrate snacks. Over-restricting treats can lead to feelings of anger and isolation. Imagine being the only child at the birthday party who is not allowed to eat cake. The psychological impact of being singled out is probably more damaging than fitting a piece of cake into the meal plan for a child with diabetes.

In addition to the general dietary guidelines listed here, carbohydrate counting or the exchange system can be used to manage carbohydrate intake and distribution. A registered dietitian who is familiar with both pediatrics and diabetes can help to develop an individualized meal plan. In the meantime, if you'd like to get started, read chapter 6 for information on carbohydrate counting and the use of exchange lists. To determine an appropriate amount of carbohydrate to strive for, you'll first need to choose an approximate calorie range. Different formulas are used to assess caloric requirements in children versus in adults. You may calculate calorie goals for adolescents who are older than age 15 by using the adult formulas included in chapter 4. Or, you may use the following formula for roughly estimating caloric requirements in youths.

Estimating Calorie Needs for Children

Start with 1,000 calories:

> add 100 calories for every year of age for females
>
> add 125 calories for every year of age for males

Examples: Maria is 13 years old. Her approximate calorie requirements are 2,300 calories per day. Peter is 16 years old. His approximated calorie requirements are 3,000 calories per day.

Kids have relatively higher calorie requirements than adults because of growth, development, and activity. The previous calculation may overestimate calorie requirements for some children, particularly older adolescents. The best way to assess your child's caloric requirements is to meet with a registered dietitian who can use your child's current height, weight, age, activity level, and diet history to determine appropriate calorie goals.

Physical Activity

Exercise is important for everyone, children as well as adults. Regular exercise is a key treatment for type 2 diabetes. Its benefits are many.

- Exercise burns glucose, so it helps to lower the blood sugar.
- Exercise burns fat, so it helps with weight control.
- Exercise makes the body's insulin work better. It decreases insulin resistance.
- Physical fitness is important for overall health and well-being.

Children should be encouraged to partake in regular physical activities. Allow them to choose activities they enjoy. Spend family time engaged in exercise. It's a wonderful way to spend quality time together. Exercising together is a lot more interactive than watching television together. Take family walks. Ride bikes together. (Remember to wear safety helmets!) Play tennis. Shoot hoops. Exercise benefits everyone. The goal should be to accumulate at least 30 minutes of physical activity each day. Beginners may choose to start with 15 minutes, 3 days per week. Then, gradually work up to the goal of at least 30 minutes per day (or more), at least 5 days per week. Here are a few more tips:

- Participate in gym classes at school.
- Join after-school team sports.
- Look into community activity programs in your area.
- Set limits on idle time spent watching TV, playing electronic games, or using computers.

See chapter 10 for more ideas and information on exercise.

Medications

When healthful meal planning and regular exercise fail to adequately control the blood sugar, medications should be added. Most pills (oral agents) used for diabetes treatment have not had clinical trials to assess safety and dosing specifically for children. Despite lack of FDA approval for use with children, oral agents are often used successfully to treat children with diabetes. (Glucophage is one oral agent that has been approved for use in children age 10 or older. Glucophage XR has been approved for use in adolescents who are age 17 or older.)

Some children with type 2 diabetes may need insulin. Insulin is FDA-approved for use by children. If children must take insulin to control blood sugar, this doesn't mean they have type 1 diabetes. Type 1 diabetes and type 2 diabetes are different diseases, with different causes. Children with type 2 diabetes may need insulin at some point and then may switch to pills at another time. Medications are often changed, reduced, or discontinued as diet, exercise, and weight control measures are established.

Support Systems

Dealing with type 2 diabetes can be especially challenging for an adolescent. Adolescents need support, and at the same time they struggle for independence. They want to fit in but must accept and cope with a chronic disease. Diabetes requires planning and many self-care strategies to prevent complications. Yet children live in the moment, tend to experiment, and generally feel invincible.

Overweight children are often teased, which can damage self-esteem. Children who have a hard time fitting in with their peers may not want to disclose that they have diabetes. Children who get chronic diseases may harbor feelings that they caused the diabetes because they did something wrong or because they were bad. Children with diabetes often experience a myriad of emotions, including anger, frustration, denial, fear, depression, and anxiety.

> There's room to fit a candy bar or a couple of cookies into the meal plan. Besides, if you don't negotiate inclusion of some favored items, those items tend to get eaten anyway. The kids just don't tell you.

Children need support. Seek the help of a counselor or mental health specialist who can meet with the child, as well as with other members of the family.

Parents can be supportive by talking with and listening to their children. Keep the lines of communication open. Provide options to children whenever possible. For example, children have to check their blood sugar. Monitoring is not an option. But you can allow the child to choose which finger to use. Remind older children that it's time to check the blood sugar but don't nag. Older children may not want their parents looking over their shoulder while the blood sugar check is being performed. But parents should have access to knowing what the numbers are. Blood sugar monitors retain a record of past readings.

> Overweight children are often teased, which can damage self-esteem. Children who have a hard time fitting in with their peers may not want to disclose that they have diabetes.

Parents should encourage physical activity and exercise. Set limits on sedentary time spent idly in front of the television, hand-held electronic games, and the computer. One of the best ways to provide support is to assist a child in following a healthful meal plan. That includes buying appropriate foods, preparing healthful meals, and measuring portions to provide the correct amount of carbohydrate and calories. Children with diabetes should not be singled out to eat entirely different foods from the rest of the family.

If diabetes camps are available in your area, children should be encouraged to attend them. Both day-camp programs and overnight camping programs can be a wonderful experience. Camps encourage healthful eating behaviors and physical activity. Diabetes self-care is a routine part of the camp experience. Children enjoy being with other children who also have diabetes. There is a sense of relief, acceptance, and camaraderie when children realize they're not alone in having diabetes. Oftentimes camp counselors and staff members have diabetes, too, and these adults provide role models for children with diabetes.

Tip: For a complete directory of diabetes camps in the United States, call the American Diabetes Association at 1-800-232-3472.

Children must learn that having diabetes doesn't have to be a roadblock in life. Children with diabetes can do anything, and be anything. They should be encouraged to believe that they are capable of attaining their goals. The sky is the limit.

Parents need support, too. Some medical clinics or communities offer support groups. If no support group is located in your area, you might consider starting one.

Diabetes in the School Setting

Children with diabetes have the right to receive care and education without discrimination. Section 504 of the Rehabilitation Act of 1973, the Individuals with Disabilities Education Act of 1991, and the Americans with Disabilities Act of 1992 are all federal laws that protect the rights of children with diabetes. Schools and day-care centers cannot discriminate against children with diabetes. Any federally funded school or any public school must accommodate the special needs of a child with diabetes, while allowing the child to participate fully in all school activities. If your school does not comply, you should file a complaint with your state's department of education.

The School's Responsibilities

- Children must be allowed to monitor their blood sugar. An appropriate location must be available if the child wants privacy. The school must assign a designated adult to assist in blood sugar monitoring if the child needs assistance.

- Medication administration must be allowed. The school must provide a safe storage site for insulin or pills that are used to treat the diabetes.

- The school must have a responsible adult available to ensure that meal and snack schedules are adhered to.

- Classroom instructors and gym teachers must be trained to watch for signs of low blood sugar in children who are treated with medications that can cause hypoglycemia. The supervising adults must know how to treat low blood sugar appropriately.

- If a child uses insulin, there must be a designated adult on the premises who is trained to administer glucagon in the event of severe low blood sugar.

- Children with diabetes must be allowed access to water/fluids as needed.

- Children with diabetes must be allowed free access to use the restroom.

- Children must be allowed to miss school without consequence to go to their doctors' appointments.

The Family's Responsibilities

- The parents should meet with school officials prior to the beginning of the school year, to find out the school's policies on diabetes.

- Parents should educate the teachers, nurse, and principal regarding their child's needs.

- Parents must ensure that a blood glucose meter is available for use at school.

- Parents should provide a list of contact numbers and instructions on whom to call in case of an emergency.

- Parents should provide a supply of appropriate items (juice, glucose tablets, snacks, glucagon) that can be used to treat low blood sugar (if the child is on medications that can cause hypoglycemia).

Preventing Type 2 Diabetes in Children

The combination of insulin resistance and decreased insulin production is an inherited disorder. Inheriting the risk of developing type 2 diabetes doesn't necessarily mean that a child will get diabetes. Usually, some other risk factors are required. Obesity and lack of physical activity are key ingredients in developing type 2 diabetes. It's important that children learn healthful eating habits, engage in regular exercise, and avoid excessive weight gain. Curbing the epidemic of obesity will require a public health approach. Schools and community programs should focus education on healthful eating behaviors and promotion of physical activity.

If a child is at high risk for developing type 2 diabetes, be sure to have that child screened every two years.

Book List

The following books can be obtained from the American Diabetes Association and may be helpful resources for parents, care providers, or teachers.

Children with Diabetes: Information for Teachers and Child-Care Providers. Alexandria, VA: American Diabetes Association, 1996.

Your School and Your Rights: Discrimination Against Children with Diabetes in the Public School System. Alexandria, VA: American Diabetes Association, 1996.

High or Low Blood Sugar. First Things First series. Alexandria, VA: American Diabetes Association, 1998.

Raising a Child with Diabetes: A Guide for Parents. Alexandria, VA: American Diabetes Association, 1995.

The Ten Keys to Helping Your Child Grow Up with Diabetes. Alexandria, VA: American Diabetes Association, 1997.

CHAPTER 14

Diabetes in Pregnancy: Twice As Important

❧

IN THIS CHAPTER

- The difference between type 2 diabetes in pregnancy and gestational diabetes
- Why tight blood sugar control is critically important
- Planning your pregnancy
- Once you are pregnant
- After the baby is born

P regnancy is a wondrous and exciting time. It's a time of change, both physically and emotionally. With the proper attention and prenatal medical care, most women with diabetes can enjoy their pregnancies and welcome a healthy baby into their lives. The importance of diabetes self-care takes on a new dimension: Caring for your diabetes translates to taking care of your developing baby.

Diabetes control throughout your pregnancy will take daily diligence. In some ways, nine months may seem like an eternity. It helps if you focus on the coming attraction. Decorate the baby's room. Think about what you'll name your baby. Accumulate baby paraphernalia. Tune in to those tiny kicks and movements within your belly. And remember, you're working hard at controlling your blood sugar for your own and your baby's benefit. Before you know it, nine months will have passed and you'll be gazing into the eyes of your new baby. All of your hard work will have been worth it.

The Difference Between Type 2 Diabetes in Pregnancy and Gestational Diabetes

Gestational diabetes is the kind of diabetes that shows up for the first time when you are pregnant and typically goes away after the baby is born. Type 2 diabetes doesn't go away after delivery.

Women are routinely tested for gestational diabetes between their 24th and 28th week of pregnancy. The hormones of pregnancy cause insulin resistance, and, in the latter part of pregnancy, a woman's pancreas has to secrete two to three times more insulin than in the pre-pregnant state. If the woman's pancreas can't step up to meet this demand, she develops elevated blood sugar during pregnancy, or gestational diabetes. Once the baby is born, the hormones return to normal levels, insulin demands concurrently drop, and the diabetes goes away. Gestational diabetes is likely to return in subsequent pregnancies. Women with gestational diabetes are at increased risk for developing type 2 diabetes at some future date. The best prevention is lifelong weight control and regular physical activity.

> With the proper attention and prenatal medical care, most women with diabetes can enjoy their pregnancies and welcome a healthy baby into their lives.

Whether a woman starts out with type 2 diabetes or develops gestational diabetes during her pregnancy, the information in this chapter is applicable.

Tip: Some women may benefit from being screened for gestational diabetes earlier than 24–28 weeks. Women with a strong family history of diabetes, women who are overweight, women who have had gestational diabetes in previous pregnancies, or women who take medications that cause insulin resistance (including medications to treat pre-term labor) should inquire about earlier screening.

Why Tight Blood Sugar Control Is Critically Important

If you have type 2 diabetes, blood sugar control is important from the first week of pregnancy all the way until you deliver your baby. The very early weeks of pregnancy are when the baby's vital organs form. Uncontrolled blood sugar during the first two to three months of pregnancy increases the risk of miscarriage and birth defects. Many women don't realize that they're pregnant until six or more weeks into the pregnancy. That's why it's critically important for women who have type 2 diabetes to achieve tight blood sugar control prior to conception. (Women don't develop gestational diabetes until later in pregnancy, which means their babies don't share these early pregnancy risks.)

Later in the pregnancy, uncontrolled blood sugar levels can cause the baby to get too big (it's called macrosomia). Think of it this way: When your blood sugar is high, the extra sugar crosses the placenta and the baby gets too many calories. Big babies are harder to deliver. The baby's shoulders can get caught in the birth canal. If the baby gets too big or the pregnancy becomes complicated, then you may need to have a cesarean section. (C-section deliveries are considered major surgery for the mother.) Very high blood sugar levels can increase the risk of stillbirth.

Another complication related to uncontrolled blood sugar is an increased risk of the mother developing preeclampsia (a serious medical condition that can result in very high blood pressure, extreme fluid retention, and loss of protein in the urine).

Uncontrolled maternal blood sugar increases the following risks to the baby: Excessive amounts of amniotic fluid can accumulate during the pregnancy, the baby's blood sugar can drop too low shortly after delivery, and the newborn may develop jaundice (temporary yellowing of the skin).

Because of all these increased risks, home deliveries are not typically recommended for women with any form of diabetes.

It will take hard work on your part, but your pregnancy can be a positive, safe, rewarding, and wonderful experience. But it takes planning.

Planning Your Pregnancy

Many women find that planning for a pregnancy brings a new wave of motivation for taking care of themselves and their diabetes. Part of planning for your pregnancy is lining up your health-care team. See your diabetes doctor, nurse educator, and dietitian and let them know that you are planning to conceive. Find an obstetrician who is familiar with high-risk pregnancies. Your health-care team can provide you with the support and information you need.

If you have preexisting complications from your diabetes, pregnancy could make them worse. Blood volume and blood pressure changes that occur during pregnancy can worsen retinopathy (eye damage), nephropathy (kidney damage), and diseases of the blood vessels or heart. Have a full medical exam before you get pregnant, and be sure to have your eyes assessed by an ophthalmologist (it's painless). A simple urine test can assess kidney health. Have a thyroid exam, breast exam, and pelvic exam.

It's important to achieve tight blood sugar control before becoming pregnant. Many health-care providers suggest at least three to six months of stable blood sugar control prior to attempting to conceive. That means using reliable contraception until you achieve tight control. Your HbA1c (hemoglobin A1c is a blood test that reflects your overall blood sugar control over the previous three months) should be within 1 percentage point above the normal, non-diabetic range. For many labs, that would mean your HbA1c should be 7 percent, or less.

If you take diabetes pills, consult with your doctor about switching to insulin prior to becoming pregnant. Oral agents are not recommended for use in pregnancy, but insulin is FDA approved for use in pregnancy. Also, make sure that any prescription drugs or over-the-counter medications that you take are safe for pregnancy.

The diet and exercise tips contained in this chapter can be started as part of your prenatal planning. Be sure to take a vitamin supplement containing 400 micrograms of folic acid as part of your pre-pregnancy plan. Then once you become pregnant, take 600 micrograms of folic acid throughout your pregnancy. Folic acid greatly reduces the risk of birth defects to the brain and spinal cord.

Tip: It's recommended that all women of childbearing age routinely take 400 micrograms of folic acid per day as a measure to protect against birth defects in the event of an unplanned pregnancy.

Tip: Prenatal vitamins are high in iron. The amount of iron in prenatal vitamins is important once you become pregnant, but during the pre-pregnancy period, a regular multivitamin is fine.

It's alright to work on weight loss prior to becoming pregnant (if you're overweight to begin with). Once you are pregnant, you shouldn't try to lose weight. Pre-pregnancy is a great time to get your exercise habits in place, too.

> The very early weeks of pregnancy are when the baby's vital organs form. Uncontrolled blood sugar during the first two to three months of pregnancy increases the risk of miscarriage and birth defects.

Once You Are Pregnant
Blood Sugar Targets

Blood sugar levels during pregnancy must be strictly controlled to reduce risks to both your baby and yourself. The closer your blood sugar is to normal, the better. The only way to track what the blood sugar is doing is to monitor your blood sugar regularly. You will likely need to check more often during pregnancy than you did prior to pregnancy.

Blood sugar levels tend to rise with each passing month of pregnancy. Increasing hormone levels are to blame. Don't stop checking your blood sugar even if the values are initially on target. Things can change. If you observe an upward trend in your readings, promptly contact your health-care team.

There are basically two types of blood glucose meters. One type of meter reports the number as a "whole blood" reading. The other type of meter reports the number as a "plasma" reading. (Plasma readings are about 11 percent higher than whole blood readings.) If you're not sure about your meter, you can call the company to inquire. The phone number should be listed on the back of your meter. Ask your team what your blood sugar targets should be. (For more information on blood sugar monitoring, see chapter 2.)

Typical Blood Sugar Targets During Pregnancy

Fasting blood sugar:

Less than or equal to 95 mg/dl if your meter reads "whole blood."

Less than or equal to 105 mg/dl if your meter reads "plasma."

Blood sugar level measured 1 hour after the meal:

Less than or equal to 140 mg/dl if your meter reads "whole blood."

Less than or equal to 155 mg/dl if your meter reads "plasma."

> It's important to achieve tight blood sugar control before becoming pregnant. Many health-care providers suggest at least three to six months of stable blood sugar control prior to attempting to get pregnant.

Caution: It's also important to prevent low blood sugar if you take insulin. See chapter 17 for more information on hypoglycemia.

Women are usually asked to check their blood sugar a minimum of four times per day: fasting (first thing in the morning, no food for the previous 8 hours) and 1 hour after each main meal (breakfast, lunch, and dinner). Women who use insulin are also asked to check their blood sugar before injecting, because their recommended insulin dose may vary according to their blood sugar level. Insulin users should also check their blood sugar any time low blood sugar is suspected. *Follow your doctor's recommendations on frequency of blood sugar monitoring and blood sugar targets.*

Weight Gain Goals

Gaining the appropriate amount of weight is an important factor in the outcome of your pregnancy. Gaining too little weight or gaining too much weight can cause problems for both the baby and you. Women who begin their pregnancy at a reasonable weight are encouraged to gain 25–35 pounds. Determine your weight gain goals based on the information in table 14.1.

Women who are short in stature are encouraged to gain at the lower end of the recommended range. Pregnancy is not the right time for weight loss, even if you start out overweight. Weight loss indicates that you don't have enough fuel, and your baby relies on you for his or her fuel. You may cringe at the thought of gaining weight, especially if you've spent much of your life trying to control it. You may feel better about a pregnancy weight gain if you know where that weight is going (see table 14.2).

Dietary Guidelines

Calories, Carbs, Protein, Fat, Fiber, and Sodium

Calorie Goals

The baby grows rapidly during the second and third trimesters of pregnancy (weeks 17–40). That's when your nutritional requirements increase by roughly 300 calories per day. A balanced diet is always

Table 14.1   Weight Gain Goals Based on Pre-Pregnancy Weight

Pre-Pregnancy Weight Class	Weight Gain Recommendation
Underweight	28–40 pounds
Average weight	25–35 pounds
Overweight	15–25 pounds
Very overweight	15 pounds

Table 14.2   Where the Weight Goes
(Values Are Approximates)

Maternal blood volume increases	1.5–4 pounds
Uterus muscle	1.5–2.5 pounds
Placenta	1–1.5 pounds
Amniotic fluid	1.5–2 pounds
Baby	7.5 pounds (varies)
Breast tissue	1–3 pounds
Maternal fat stores	0–10 pounds (varies)

important. But don't start "eating for two" in the first couple of months of your pregnancy, or you may end up gaining too much weight.

Tip: A normal pregnancy lasts 40 weeks. The first trimester is considered weeks 1–16, the second trimester is weeks 17–35, and the third trimester is week 36 to delivery.

To determine your calorie goals during pregnancy, first assess your nonpregnant calorie goals using chapter 4, then add 300 calories per day during months 4–9. Most women end up needing a total of about 2,000–2,200 calories per day (your needs may vary). Monitor your weight. Calorie goals should be adjusted to ensure appropriate weight gain.

A minimum of 1,700–1,800 calories per day is recommended during pregnancy. Eating too few calories or too few carbohydrates can cause the production of ketones. Ketones are acidic byproducts that form because of a relative lack of insulin (generally in type 1 diabetes), but ketones can also form from over-restricting calories or not eating enough carbohydrate. Ketones can pass through the placenta and may have a negative impact on the fetus. You can test for ketone production by dipping a ketone test strip in your urine. Ask your health-care provider for a prescription for ketone test strips.

Carbohydrate Intake Recommendations

Diabetes during pregnancy is one situation when a slightly lower carbohydrate intake may be prudent. I usually recommend that 40–50 percent of the calories come from carbohydrate (see table 14.3). Higher carbohydrate intake may make it difficult to maintain the strict blood sugar control required during pregnancy. It's equally important to ensure adequate carbohydrate intake. If you eat too little carbohydrate, then important nutrients from the carbohydrate food groups may be lacking. Grains, milk, and fruits are each important components of a healthful diet. I've met too many women who have over-restricted their intake of carbohydrate foods in hopes of controlling their blood sugar levels. Don't lose sight of the big picture. Growing a healthy baby requires a balanced, healthful diet. The hormones of pregnancy can cause your blood sugar to go too high even when you eat appropriately. If that's the case, administering insulin—not over-restricting your diet—is the likely solution.

> Pregnancy is not the right time for weight loss, even if you start out overweight. Weight loss indicates that you don't have enough fuel, and your baby relies on you for his or her fuel.

Tip: If you take insulin, you may be able to tolerate a somewhat higher carbohydrate intake, because the insulin dose can be adjusted to accommodate it.

Once you determine your carbohydrate goals, it's important to distribute your carbohydrate intake throughout the day. Eating too much at one time can cause the blood sugar to go dangerously high. It works best to split your carbohydrate budget between three meals and two to three snacks—for example, 45–60 grams of carbohydrate for each main meal (3–4 carbohydrate exchanges) and 15–30 grams of carbohydrate for each snack (1–2 carbohydrate exchanges). Adjust according to your carbohydrate intake goals.

Tip: Use whole grains, brown rice, and fresh fruits and vegetables to increase your fiber intake.

Table 14.3 Providing 40–50 Percent of Calories As Carbohydrate

Calorie Level	Daily Grams of Carbohydrate	Number of Carbohydrate Exchanges
1,700	170–213	11–14
1,800	180–225	12–15
1,900	190–238	13–16
2,000	200–250	13–17
2,100	210–263	14–18
2,200	220–275	15–18
2,300	230–288	15–19
2,400	240–300	16–20
2,500	250–313	17–21
2,600	260–325	17–22

Protein Intake Recommendations

Pregnancy increases your protein requirements. Protein is required to build blood cells and tissues for both the mother and the fetus. Daily protein intake should be at least 60 grams. Protein should supply roughly 20–25 percent of your total calories (see table 14.4). However, your protein recommendations may vary according to preexisting medical conditions. It's not necessary to count grams of protein every day, but you should do a rough assessment of your average protein intake to ensure adequacy.

Tip: Given the higher protein intake recommended with pregnancy, it is especially important to choose lean selections of meat and nonfat or lowfat dairy products.

Table 14.4   Providing 20–25 Percent of Calories As Protein

Calorie Level	Daily Grams of Protein Recommended
1,700	85–106
1,800	90–113
1,900	95–119
2,000	100–125
2,100	105–131
2,200	110–138
2,300	115–144
2,400	120–150
2,500	125–156
2,600	130–163

Fat Intake Recommendations

Fats should be approximately 25–35 percent of your intake, depending on your chosen carbohydrate and protein goals (see table 14.5). It's not necessary to count grams of fat every day. However, if you're gaining weight too rapidly, take a critical look at how much fat you eat. Reducing fat intake can slow the rate of weight gain.

Tip: As always, choose heart-healthy fats and oils most of the time. Some of the best choices are olive oil, canola oil, peanut oil, olives, avocados, peanuts, walnuts, and fresh fish.

Fiber Recommendations

Recommended intake for fiber during pregnancy is the same as for nonpregnant adults; 20–35 grams per day from a combination of foods.

**Table 14.5   Providing 25–35 Percent of Calories
As Fat**

Calorie Level	Daily Grams of Fat Recommended
1,700	47–66
1,800	50–70
1,900	53–74
2,000	56–78
2,100	58–82
2,200	61–86
2,300	64–89
2,400	67–93
2,500	69–97
2,600	72–101

Fiber can help to prevent and treat constipation. To best ensure an adequate intake of fiber, it's suggested that you eat at least five portions per day from a combination of fruits and vegetables, as well as at least six servings per day from the grains and starch group. Try to include more whole grains, and less refined grain products. Be sure to drink plenty of fluids when increasing your fiber intake. To review fiber content of select foods, see chapter 18.

Sodium Recommendations

Recommended sodium intake during pregnancy is the same as for nonpregnant adults: less than 3,000 milligrams per day. (Americans typically consume 4,000–8,000 mg each day.) For women with high

blood pressure, sodium intake should be limited to somewhere between 2,000–2,400 milligrams per day.

Mild swelling of the feet, ankles, and hands is a common occurrence
during pregnancy. Changing hormone levels are to blame for the puffi-
ness. Pregnancy-related mild fluid retention does not warrant sodium
restriction. Severe fluid retention, especially if accompanied by headache, nausea, or visual changes, may signal a much more serious condition
known as preeclampsia, which requires swift medical attention.

Dietary Strategies for Controlling the Blood Sugar

- Distribute your foods between three meals and two to three
  snacks. Distributing the carbohydrate throughout the day allows
  your body to process it one batch at a time. Smaller, more
  frequent meals help to ensure that your blood sugar doesn't go
  too high after a meal.

- Milk and fruit are both healthful
  choices. However, they tend to digest
  rather quickly, which means that the
  glucose derived from those foods
  enters the bloodstream rapidly. To
  prevent spiking post-meal blood sugar
  levels, it's recommended to eat those
  foods one portion at a time. In other
  words, if you're striving for 45–60

  > A balanced diet is always important. But don't start "eating for two" in the first couple of months of your pregnancy, or you may end up gaining too much weight.

  grams of carbohydrate per meal, don't spend your entire carbohydrate budget on a fruit platter. It's fine to have three to four
  portions of fruit per day, but one per meal or snack. The same
  goes for milk.

- Avoid fruit juice, even if it's home-squeezed, 100 percent natural
  juice. It just raises the blood sugar too much. Avoid regular soft
  drinks and sugary beverages. Blood sugar levels during pregnancy must stay in tight control. (It's acceptable to use juice to
  treat low blood sugar reactions caused by insulin.)

- Avoid added sugars. That includes natural sugars, honey, and syrups. You can't afford to waste your carbohydrate budget on non-nutritious foods. Every bite should count toward good nutrition. Besides, concentrated sweets can cause your blood sugar to rise too much. Fit your favorite treats into your meal plan after your baby is born.

- Blood sugar levels can be especially difficult to control at breakfast time. That's because hormone levels tend to make you more insulin-resistant in the mornings, which means your insulin doesn't work as well at controlling your blood sugar. If your blood sugar monitoring shows that your post-breakfast blood sugar values are creeping up, try to skip the milk and fruit at the breakfast meal (since those foods digest so quickly). Eat them, but eat them at meals or snacks other than breakfast. A breakfast that consists of starch plus protein may be better tolerated. Another option is to limit breakfast to 30 grams of carbohydrate and distribute the remaining carbohydrate between the other meals and snacks. But *don't* skip breakfast.

Vital Vitamins and Mighty Minerals

Folic Acid

Folic acid (folate) is a B vitamin that is crucial during the first few weeks of pregnancy. Folic acid greatly reduces the risk of certain birth defects, known as neural tube defects, which affect the spine and the brain of the developing fetus and can occur before a woman even knows that she's pregnant. The recommended daily allowance (RDA) for folic acid during pregnancy is 600 micrograms per day. Ideally, supplementation should begin before conception. (All women of childbearing age should consume at least 400 micrograms of folic acid per day.) Check the label on your multivitamin to ensure that it supplies sufficient amounts

> Pregnancy increases your protein requirements. Protein is required to build blood cells and tissues for both the mother and the fetus.

of folic acid. The RDA for breastfeeding is 500 micrograms per day. Many breakfast cereals and grain products are fortified with folic acid. Folic acid is also found in legumes (dried beans), wheat germ, and dark green leafy vegetables.

Vitamin B12

Vitamin B12, along with folate, is needed to produce new blood cells. Pregnancy is a time when maternal blood volume increases dramatically. Vitamin B12 is important in preventing anemia and is needed to produce maternal and fetal tissues. Vitamin B12 is relatively easy to obtain in a balanced diet. In fact, B12 is found in all animal products, including milk, cheese, yogurt, meat, fish, poultry, and eggs. Strict vegetarians who omit all animal products must take a vitamin B12 supplement. The RDA for pregnancy is 2.6 micrograms per day. The RDA for breastfeeding is 2.8 micrograms per day.

Vitamin A

Vitamin A is essential for growth and development of the fetus. It's also important for normal vision and a healthy immune system. (The immune system battles infections.) The RDA for vitamin A in pregnancy is 770 micrograms per day, except for women 18 years or younger, who should get 750 micrograms per day. The RDA for breastfeeding is 1,300 micrograms per day, except for women 18 years or younger, who should get 1,200 micrograms per day.

Tip: Vitamin A is listed several different ways on a label:

1 IU is the same as 0.3 micrograms.

1 microgram is the same as 1 RAE, or 1 RE.

Caution: Do not exceed the RDA for vitamin A without medical supervision. High intake of vitamin A has been linked to birth defects and miscarriage. (Beta-carotene, the precursor to vitamin A that is found in dark yellow and dark orange fruits and vegetables, does *not* carry these risks. For reference, 1 microgram or 1 RAE of vitamin A is equal to 12 micrograms of beta-carotene.)

Iron

Iron is a mineral that is needed for the production of red blood cells, as well as maternal and fetal tissues. The RDA for iron during pregnancy is set at 27 milligrams per day. Prenatal vitamins supply at least this level of iron. For women who develop anemia during pregnancy, iron doses of 60 milligrams per day are often recommended. The RDAs for breastfeeding drop to 9 milligrams per day, except for women 18 years or younger, who should get 10 milligrams per day. Major dietary sources of iron include organ meats, red meat, poultry, seafood (especially clams, oysters, and mussels), legumes (dried beans), dark green leafy vegetables, and enriched cereals and grains.

Tip: Don't take iron supplements at the same time as calcium supplements. Iron and calcium can bind together and inhibit each other's absorption. Don't take iron supplements with calcium-rich dairy products for the same reason.

Tip: Iron can cause constipation. Be sure to drink plenty of water and to eat a diet rich in fiber to help prevent and treat constipation.

Zinc

Zinc is a mineral that is important for synthesis of new tissue. The RDA for zinc during pregnancy is 11 milligrams per day (13 milligrams per day for women aged 18 or younger). The RDA for breastfeeding is 12 milligrams per day (14 milligrams per day for women aged 18 or younger). Dietary sources of zinc include meat, liver, seafood (especially oysters), eggs, whole grains, and wheat germ.

Calcium

Calcium is a mineral that is needed to form bones and teeth. If you don't get enough calcium, you may deplete some of the calcium from your own bones to provide the baby with calcium. Avoid the calcium tug-of-war. Make sure you get enough calcium for both yourself and your baby. Dairy products are the best source of calcium. Strive for 3–4 portions of milk, yogurt, or cheese each day. Nondairy options include calcium-fortified tofu or calcium-fortified soy milk. The RDA for calcium during pregnancy and breastfeeding is 1,000 milligrams per day. Young moms who are 18 years or younger when they get pregnant need more calcium. They should strive for 1,300 milligrams per day because their own bones are still absorbing calcium. Insufficient calcium intake can weaken your bone structure and increases the risk of developing osteoporosis later in life.

Tip: To control weight gain, choose nonfat or lowfat dairy products.

Tip: Don't take calcium supplements at the same time as iron supplements or with your prenatal vitamin. Calcium and iron can bind together and inhibit each other's absorption. Also, if you take more than one calcium tablet per day, don't take them all at the same time. You'll absorb more of the calcium supplement if you space the dose out through the day—for example, 500 milligrams with lunch and 500 milligrams with dinner instead of 1,000 milligrams all together.

> The hormones of pregnancy can cause your blood sugar to go too high even when you eat appropriately. If that's the case, administering insulin—not over-restricting your diet—is the likely solution.

Common Dietary Concerns

Caffeine

Less is better. A large intake of caffeine may pose significant risks to the developing fetus. Do without, if you can. If not, limit your caffeine intake to one caffeinated beverage per day.

Alcoholic Beverages

All alcoholic beverages should be completely avoided during pregnancy. Alcohol exposure is harmful to the fetus. Alcohol can cause birth defects and mental retardation in the baby.

Artificial Sweeteners

The FDA has approved the safety of using the following artificial sweeteners during pregnancy:

Aspartame

Acesulfame-K

Sucralose

See chapter 16 for more information on artificial sweeteners.

Tips for Digestive Discomforts

Morning Sickness

I'm not sure why they call it morning sickness. I had it morning, noon, and night. Most women suffer some degree of nausea or vomiting during their pregnancy. It usually resolves around the third or fourth month. Others have a more persistent and severe disorder known as hyperemesis gravidarum, which is severe vomiting that requires medical intervention.

Tips for Nausea and Vomiting

- Eat small, frequent meals (nausea is usually worse when your stomach is empty).

- Try dry, bland starches such as toast or crackers.

- Try cold foods. They have fewer odors and may be less offensive.

- Limit greasy, fatty, or fried foods.

- Avoid the specific foods that bother you.

- Ask someone else to help with food preparation.

- Keep the kitchen and dining room ventilated with fresh air.

- Try ginger tea (make by boiling 1 inch of fresh ginger root, minced, to 2 cups of water).

Heartburn

As the baby grows and presses on your stomach, the contents of the stomach can be pushed up through the top opening of the stomach and into the esophagus, causing stomach acids to burn the tender tissue of the esophagus. It helps to eat smaller, more frequent meals.

Tips to Minimize the Symptoms of Heartburn

- Avoid greasy, fatty, or fried foods.
- Eliminate spicy foods if they bother you.
- Drink your fluids between meals, rather than with meals.
- Don't lie down after a meal.
- Wear loose-fitting clothes.
- Avoid caffeine.
- Eat slowly.

Constipation

Pregnancy hormones cause food to move through the intestines more slowly. Iron supplements can add to the woes of constipation. If you incorporate all of the tips here and still suffer from constipation, tell your health-care provider. Medications are available to relieve constipation.

Tips for Constipation

- Drink plenty of fluids (8–10 cups of noncaffeinated fluid per day).
- Increase your fiber intake by using whole grains.
- Increase your fiber intake by including fresh fruits and plenty of vegetables.
- If you use prunes, limit to three prunes because of the high sugar content in dried fruits.
- Include regular exercise (which brings me to the next topic . . .).

Exercise

The Benefits of Exercise During Pregnancy

Exercise has many health benefits. Most women can, and should, partake in mild to moderate exercise during their pregnancies. In addition to the many health benefits discussed in chapter 10, exercise has specific benefits during pregnancy.

- Exercise helps to control blood sugar levels.

- Exercise improves strength and stamina.

- Exercise helps your body prepare for labor and delivery.

- Exercise may help to prevent excessive weight gain.

- Exercise helps to prevent and treat constipation.

- Exercise improves fitness and relieves back pain.

- Exercise improves your mood, relieves stress, and helps you to sleep better.

> Alcohol exposure is harmful to the fetus. Alcohol can cause birth defects and mental retardation in the baby.

Safety First

Discuss your exercise plan with your health-care provider. Certain medical conditions, pregnancy complications, or preexisting diabetes complications may impose exercise restrictions. Find out if you have any medical or pregnancy-related exercise limitations and follow your doctor's advice.

Monitor your blood sugar before and after exercise to see how you respond to activity. If you take insulin, be sure to carry a carbohydrate-containing snack in case your blood sugar drops. Drink plenty of water. Exercise, pregnancy, and diabetes all increase your fluid requirements.

Just as exercise has benefits unique to pregnancy, certain safety issues are unique to exercising during pregnancy. Here are some pointers:

- As your abdomen expands, your center of gravity will change. This will affect your balance and posture. Watch your step.

- Pregnancy hormones cause tendons and ligaments to loosen and stretch, which can increase your chances of exercise-related injury. Avoid abrupt, jerky motions. Remember to warm up before your exercise session and to cool down at the end of your session.

- Pregnancy causes a significant increase in blood volume. Your heart's workload increases. You may notice that you get winded quicker. Don't overdo it.

- Your heart rate shouldn't exceed 140 beats per minute.

- You're more likely to become short of breath as your body's oxygen demands change. Don't exercise to the point of exhaustion. If you're short of breath, you may be compromising oxygen delivery to your baby. Stop and catch your breath.

- Don't take risks. Avoid activities that could cause trauma to the abdomen.

- Avoid exercises that compress the abdomen.

- Avoid exercises that involve bouncy, jumping motions.

- As your belly enlarges, avoid exercises that require you to lie flat on your back. That position is associated with a decrease in blood flow and oxygen delivery to the baby.

> Higher carbohydrate intake may make it difficult to maintain the strict blood sugar control required during pregnancy. It's equally important to ensure adequate carbohydrate intake. If you eat too little carbohydrate, then important nutrients from the carbohydrate food groups may be lacking. Grains, milk, and fruits are each important components of a healthful diet.

Caution! STOP exercising and call your doctor:

- If you experience significant shortness of breath or pain

- If you notice changes in your vision

- If you feel dizzy, lightheaded, or get a headache

- If you begin leaking fluid or bleeding vaginally

- If you experience contractions that could indicate pre-term labor

- For any reason that *you* feel is significant

Reasons to Avoid Exercise During Pregnancy

- If you are bleeding vaginally or leaking fluid

- If your bag of waters has broken

- If you have preeclampsia (severe high blood pressure during pregnancy)

- If your healthcare provider has advised you to avoid exercise

Tip: If you are on bedrest, ask your doctor for guidelines on allowable activities.

Medications

As the weeks of pregnancy march on, pregnancy hormones get stronger and stronger. As the hormone levels rise, the blood sugar typically gets harder to control. Don't be disheartened if you're doing everything in your power to control your blood sugar and the numbers start to creep up despite your best efforts. What worked well in the sixth month may no longer work in the eighth month. When dietary interventions and exercise fail to control the blood sugar adequately, insulin is called for. If your doctor prescribes insulin, don't despair. The needles are actually smaller than those you use to check your blood sugar. Insulin is perfectly safe. It's a natural hormone that's made by your pancreas. If your own pancreas can't keep up with the demands of pregnancy, you may need supplemental insulin. Injected insulin does not cross the placenta. Most women who start insulin therapy during pregnancy can stop taking insulin after the baby is born and hormone levels return to normal. Diabetes pills are not considered safe to take during pregnancy, as oral agents may pose risks to the baby. If you took diabetes pills before you got pregnant, you'll most likely resume taking them after your baby is born.

After the Baby Is Born

First of all, congratulations are in order! The real journey begins now! Enjoy your baby. Motherhood is very rewarding. It's also hard work. Your baby will take a lot of your attention, which is great. Just remember to pay attention to your diabetes, too.

Once the baby and placenta are delivered, maternal hormone levels return to normal. If you had been taking insulin during your pregnancy, it will likely be decreased or discontinued. Your doctor may prescribe diabetes pills if you took them prior to pregnancy.

I hope you are planning to breastfeed your infant. Breast milk is a superior choice in most situations. It's typically recommended to breastfeed through the first year of life. If for some reason you can't breastfeed for an entire year, whatever you can do is beneficial for your baby. Breast milk offers the baby important antibodies that are passed through the milk from mother to child. Antibodies help to provide immunity from illnesses that your baby is exposed to in those first months. Breast milk production uses about 500 calories per day (which can help you to lose some of the weight gained during pregnancy). It's important to continue to eat a healthful diet and make sure you get three to four servings of calcium-rich dairy products or other calcium sources that equal at least 1,000 milligrams per day (1,300 milligrams for moms aged 18 years old or under). You should also continue to take a multivitamin during your breastfeeding months. To ensure an adequate milk supply, drink plenty of fluids.

> If you take diabetes pills, consult with your doctor about switching to insulin prior to becoming pregnant. Oral agents are not recommended for use during pregnancy.

It's fine to work on weight loss once the baby has arrived, but don't over-restrict calories if you're breastfeeding. Focus on eating less fat and getting regular exercise.

For women who developed gestational diabetes during their pregnancies, it's important to have follow-up evaluation to ensure that their blood sugar levels have returned to normal. Women with gestational

diabetes stand a significant risk of developing type 2 diabetes sometime in the future and should be screened for type 2 diabetes at least
every three years, and certainly before attempting to get pregnant again.

CHAPTER 15

The Golden Years

ॐ

IN THIS CHAPTER

- Blood sugar control is important at all ages
- Diabetes in the elderly: a growing concern
- Health care
- Self-care
- Community resources

Blood Sugar Control Is Important at All Ages

Once, a 71-year-old client told me that he didn't want to be bothered with the tasks of diabetes care. He said, "I don't want to follow a diet, and I don't want to check my blood sugar. I paid my dues in life. Now I just want to enjoy myself. I don't care if it means I live a year or two less." He assumed that since he got diabetes later in life, he probably wouldn't develop major diabetic complications in his lifetime. What he hadn't considered was that his uncontrolled diabetes was affecting his current day-to-day living. He felt sluggish and had a hard time concentrating. He complained of blurry vision, so he gave up reading, which had previously been a favorite pastime. His sleep was interrupted by frequent trips to the bathroom. He had assumed that the frequent urination was because of his prostate. But in fact, his high blood sugar levels turned out to be the main culprit. Once he implemented some key dietary tips and started on the right medications, he admitted he felt much better. He also started checking his blood sugar twice a day. As his blood sugar levels improved, his vision improved and he picked up reading again.

Don't let diabetes tarnish your golden years. Having diabetes doesn't have to interfere with your ability to enjoy retirement. Don't assume that every health complaint you have is a necessary part of aging. Get a full medical evaluation. Take control of your diabetes.

The consequences of high blood sugar include:

- Fatigue and lethargy
- Increased frequency of urination
    - which can cause incontinence
    - which can interrupt sleep patterns
    - which can lead to dehydration
    - which can cause mineral deficiencies because certain minerals are lost in the urine (particularly zinc, chromium, and magnesium)
- Blurred vision (which can resolve with improved blood sugar control)
- Impotence
- Poor wound healing
- Decreased ability to fight infection
- Increased stickiness of factors in the blood (platelets), which increases the risk of heart attack and stroke
- Confusion and hallucinations, which if not promptly treated can lead to coma and death

Diabetes in the elderly is often undertreated. That is a real disservice. All too often individuals have had type 2 diabetes for many years before actually being diagnosed, which increases the risk for developing complications. Your diabetes must be effectively managed. If your health-care provider is not aggressive enough in managing your diabetes, you may want to look for a health-care provider who will be. If possible, seek the advice of a diabetes specialist: an endocrinologist.

Diabetes in the Elderly: A Growing Concern

The fastest-growing segment of the American population consists of individuals aged 60 and older. In 1994, one out of every eight individuals in our country was over 65 years old. By the year 2020 it is estimated that one out of every six people will be over 65 years old.

Approximately 20 percent of people aged 65 years or older have diabetes, and just about half of those people don't even know that they have it! Another 20 percent of people over the age of 65 have impaired glucose tolerance, which means their blood sugar levels are higher than normal but not yet high enough to be classified as diabetes. That adds up to a full 40 percent of our senior citizens with some degree of glucose intolerance! That statistic is not matched the world over. Some societies report diabetes prevalence as low as 3.5 percent in their senior populations. Advancing age is a risk factor for developing diabetes, but having 65 candles on the cake doesn't make diabetes an inevitability. Prevention strategies boil down to accessing health care and implementing self-care.

> Don't let diabetes tarnish your golden years. Having diabetes doesn't have to interfere with your ability to enjoy retirement.

Health Care
Clinic Visits

Have regular medical check-ups. Just as your trusty automobile needs an occasional tune-up, your body needs a thorough inspection to ensure that everything is in optimal working condition. See chapter 2 for the check-up checklist.

Many individuals have had diabetes for several years before finding out about it. That's why it's so important to have a thorough exam at the time of diagnosis. Be sure to get screened for possible diabetes-related problems.

- See an ophthalmologist for a dilated eye exam.

- Get your urine tested to check your kidney health.

- Have your feet examined for nerve damage and circulatory problems.

- Have your risk for heart disease assessed (heart disease is the most common disease present in senior citizens).

Tip: A complete physical exam should be done every year.

Tip: If you unintentionally gain or lose more than 10 pounds in a 6-month period, be sure to inform your health-care provider.

> All too often individuals have had type 2 diabetes for many years before actually being diagnosed, which increases the risk for developing complications.

Diabetes tune-up visits should be scheduled every three to six months. Your doctor may want to see you more or less often, depending on your health history. Have your feet inspected at every clinic visit. Take your shoes off when you get into the exam room. That way you will be sure that it gets done. Foot care is important because nerve damage and poor circulation can contribute to serious problems. Inspect your own feet every day. If it's hard for you to see your feet, use a mirror or enlist the help of someone else. Be prompt in reporting abnormalities to your doctor. A podiatrist—a doctor who specializes in foot care—can do your toenail trimming if it's hard for you to do so. Improper toenail trimming can lead to ingrown toenails or dangerous infections if tender skin gets snipped by mistake.

Blood pressure control is crucial, so you should have your blood pressure checked at every clinic visit. If you have hypertension (high blood pressure), see chapter 12 for more information.

Ask your doctor about ordering a medical alert bracelet or pendant. Wearing identification that says you have diabetes will help ensure that you get the care you need should an emergency arise.

Tip: Have your doctor refer you to a registered dietitian to plan a healthful diet for diabetes. A registered dietitian can also provide nutrition therapy advice for weight control and therapeutic diet strategies for other health issues. In addition, make sure you see a diabetes nurse educator to learn how to use a home blood sugar monitor.

Tip: When you go for diabetes education visits, consider bringing a friend or family member. You'll have twice the listening power!

Medications

More than one senior citizen has told me they feel as if they could open a pharmacy with all of the medications they take. It's not unusual to take multiple prescription drugs in your senior years. Be sure to tell each of your health-care providers about all the medications and supplements that you take (including herbs and vitamins). Some medications should not be taken together. Certain medical conditions prohibit the use of some types of diabetes medication. Be open and honest with your health-care providers. Don't hold back information. Your safety relies on it.

Many types of medication can be used to treat diabetes. Your health-care provider can choose the one that best suits you. Sometimes two or more different diabetes medications are needed to achieve adequate control. If you require insulin to control your diabetes, ask your doctor or diabetes nurse educator about devices that simplify the process. Arthritis and poor vision can make it difficult for you to draw up and mix insulin. You may benefit from using magnifying devices or pre-mixed insulin, or you may find the insulin pens a simple alternative to syringes.

Medication Tips

- Keep an updated list of your medications and doses in your wallet.

- Bring a complete list of your medications and doses to all clinic visits.

- If you have any questions about your medications, ask your doctor or a pharmacist.

- Find out what times you should take your medication.

- Find out whether your medication should be taken on an empty stomach or with food.

- Find out if you have two medications that should not be taken at the same time.

- Get a pill organizer from your local drugstore.

- If you forget a dose of medication, don't double up the next dose.

- Make sure you get refills before you get down to your last several pills.

- Don't start any medications without your doctor's approval.

- Don't discontinue any medications without your doctor's approval.

- Report any medication-related side effects to your doctor.

- If you're having bouts of hypoglycemia, ask your health-care provider to adjust your dose or to switch you to another medication that doesn't cause low blood sugar.

Self-Care
Nutritional Considerations

Does it seem as if food has lost its appeal? As you age, your sense of taste and smell may diminish. The foods that you used to love may now bore you. Some prescription medications may cause digestive complaints or leave a bad taste in your mouth. The net effect might be that you don't eat as well as you should. Many seniors are compromised nutritionally. Common problems include not eating enough and not eating the right things. Your body needs balanced nutrition now as much as ever.

Barriers to Balanced Nutrition

Besides appetite changes, social situations can contribute to malnutrition. The loss of a beloved mate can result in depression and a dwindling appetite. Cooking and eating for one just isn't the same as sharing mealtimes together. Isolation is associated with poor eating habits, and living on a fixed income can dictate the types and amounts of foods available.

Foot care is important because nerve damage and poor circulation can contribute to serious problems. Inspect your own feet every day.

In some cases, advancing age brings physical limitations that impact the ability to shop for, prepare, and eat meals. Barriers include visual problems, arthritis, ill-fitting dentures, changes in strength and balance, and decreased mobility.

Eating Tips

- Share meals with friends or family whenever possible.

- Eat a variety of foods.

- Try new recipes.

- When you cook, make extra and freeze leftovers for future use.

- Eat 5–6 small meals per day.

- Eat adequate amounts of protein (see chapter 7 for information on protein).

- Frozen vegetables can be used as needed, and they keep well.

- Unprocessed potatoes, rice, dried beans, and pastas are cheaper than prepared items.

- Eat fresh fruit, or buy fruits canned in their own juices or in water, not in syrup.

- Use foods with stronger flavors and seasonings if your sense of taste has diminished.

- Focus on using herbs and spices instead of added salt.

- Make foods look attractive.

- Set a fancy table.

- Increase fiber to treat and prevent constipation (see chapter 18 for more on fiber).

- Drink plenty of liquids.

- Keep active; it stimulates the appetite.

- If you eat at senior centers or have meals delivered to your home, ask for diabetic menu options.

Senior Nutrition Alert

Calorie requirements decrease somewhat as the years pass by, but vitamin and mineral requirements don't significantly decrease. It's important to make every bite count. Choose nutritious and fortified foods and limit junk foods.

> As you age, your sense of taste and smell may diminish. The foods that you used to love may now bore you.

As the body ages, the sense of thirst diminishes. Don't wait for thirst to tell you when to drink! One common problem affecting seniors is dehydration. Uncontrolled diabetes further increases your risk for dehydration. Adequate fluid intake is crucially important. Be sure to drink enough water. Aim for at least 8 cups of fluid per day, and drink more on hot days. (Alcoholic beverages don't count toward fluid goals.)

Tip: Ask your health-care provider if you have any medical conditions that affect your fluid goals.

If you regularly eat a well-balanced diet, you don't have to take vitamin supplements. If you choose to take a multivitamin supplement, pick one that provides 100 percent of the RDA (recommended daily allowance). The vitamin supplements are in addition to, not in place of, healthful foods.

Caution: Exceeding the RDA is not recommended because high intake of certain vitamins (especially vitamin A) can cause toxicity.

Seniors have an increased risk for deficiency in the following specific vitamins and minerals:

Vitamin B12

Decreased stomach acid secretion in many elderly individuals results in poor vitamin B12 absorption. Vitamin B12 is found in all animal products. The RDA for vitamin B12 in seniors is 2.4 micrograms per day.

Calcium

The RDA for seniors is 1,200 milligrams of calcium per day, but many seniors don't get that much. Dairy products are excellent sources of calcium. A cup of milk, a cup of yogurt, or 1½ ounces of cheese each supply about 300 milligrams of calcium. Another option is to use calcium-fortified soy milk or calcium-fortified tofu. If you don't get enough dietary calcium, you should take a calcium supplement.

Tip: If milk makes you feel bloated, gassy, or gives you diarrhea, you may be lactose intolerant (which means you lack the enzyme for digesting the milk sugar called lactose). Lactaid brand milk contains the enzymes necessary for digesting milk. Another alternative is to buy Lactaid pills or Lactaid drops at your local drugstore and take them when you drink milk.

Tip: Don't use calcium supplements that contain dolomite, aluminum, or bone meal.

Tip: Don't take calcium supplements at the same time as iron supplements because the two minerals interfere with each other's absorption.

Vitamin D

Vitamin D is necessary, along with calcium, for bone strength. Vitamin D can be made in your body by a chemical reaction that occurs when sunlight shines on your skin. Vitamin D is found in fortified milk. If you don't drink much milk and if you spend most of your time indoors, then you may not get the vitamin D you require to maintain healthy bones. The RDA for vitamin D in seniors is 10 micrograms per day if you're between 51 and 70 years old and 15 micrograms per day if you're over 70.

Tip: Vitamin D content may be listed as micrograms or international units (IU); 1 microgram is equal to 40 IU.

Vitamin C

Vitamin C is important for wound healing and improves the absorption of the iron found in green leafy vegetables and in iron supplements. Many fruits and vegetables offer vitamin C. The RDA for an adult female is 75 milligrams per day. The RDA for an adult male is 90 milligrams per day.

Zinc

Zinc is important for fighting infection and aiding in wound healing. Dietary sources include meat, liver, seafood, eggs, whole grains, wheat germ, bran, legumes, and nuts. The RDA for adult females is 8 milligrams per day. The RDA for adult males is 11 milligrams per day.

Magnesium

Magnesium is used in many chemical processes in the body. It's found in nuts, seeds, legumes (dried beans), and whole grains. The RDA for elderly females is 320 milligrams per day, and for elderly males it's 420 milligrams per day.

Folate

Folate is needed to make new cells and new tissues. Folate is abundant in leafy vegetables, legumes (dried beans), and some fruits. The RDA for elderly adults is 400 micrograms per day.

Exercise Considerations

Exercise helps with blood sugar control, blood pressure control, and cardiac fitness. Other benefits important to seniors include increased strength and endurance and retention of both muscle mass and bone density—all of which increase the ability to live independently.

Elderly individuals have a higher risk of heart problems and other physical ailments. That's why it's important to have a complete medical exam, exercise stress test, and your health-care provider's blessing before initiating an exercise program. If you have complications or certain medical conditions, your health-care provider may advise you to avoid particular types of exercise. For example, if you have diabetic eye disease, you should not strain or bear down because it increases the pressure in the eyes. Heavy weight lifting would be out of the question. Follow your doctor's advice on exercise!

> One common problem affecting seniors is dehydration. Uncontrolled diabetes further increases your risk for dehydration.

Don't forget the importance of the warm-up and cool-down periods. Start slowly, and don't overdo it. Seniors should exercise at a lower intensity than that recommended for the younger crowd.

Senior-Friendly Exercises

- Swimming and water aerobics tend to be easy on the joints.

- Walking and riding a stationary bicycle are excellent forms of exercise.

- If you're unsteady on your feet, try armchair exercises that involve leg and arm movements while you're seated in a chair.

- If you have a history of heart disease, ask for a referral to a cardiac-rehab center.

- Try a low-impact exercise video.

- Walk the inner perimeters of a shopping mall.

- Find out if your local senior center organizes exercise classes.

- Tune in to a television exercise program geared toward seniors.

- Exercises like yoga can improve flexibility and balance.

- Try weight lifting with light weights to build strength.

  See chapter 10 for more information on exercise and safety precautions.

Blood Sugar Monitoring

Checking your blood sugar is an important component of diabetes self-care. It's the only way that you can be sure your numbers are in a safe range. Ask your health-care provider what your blood sugar values should be. For the most part, blood sugar targets for seniors are the same as for younger adults. If you take a diabetes medication that could cause low blood sugar, then your doctor may set your blood sugar targets somewhat higher to prevent the risk of hypoglycemia. Low blood sugar could result in losing your balance and falling.

> Start slowly, and don't overdo it. Seniors should exercise at a lower intensity than that recommended for the younger crowd.

The frequency of blood sugar monitoring depends upon your overall diabetes control, the medications you take, and your general health. Ask your health-care provider for recommendations. A diabetes nurse educator can help you choose a meter that best suits your needs. Ask for a simple-to-use meter with a large display screen for ease in reading the numbers. Get a meter with a built-in memory. Make sure you know how to operate the meter. Don't be shy about asking for help. No one knows how to use a meter before being properly trained. Be sure to check your meter for accuracy periodically by running a control solution test. Your diabetes educator can show you how. Meters are available for the visually impaired. Bring your meter and your blood sugar logbook to all clinic appointments. (See chapter 2 for more information on blood sugar monitoring.)

Generally speaking, blood sugar values before meals should be roughly 80–120 mg/dl. Blood sugar values after meals should not exceed 180 mg/dl (some people set the target for 160 mg/dl or below), and blood sugar at bedtime should be 100–140 mg/dl. Individual goals may vary, based on whether or not you take medications or have specific health problems. Don't wait for your next scheduled clinic appointment if your blood sugar is out of control. Call your clinic and ask to be seen sooner, so that you can regain control of your diabetes.

Community Resources

Many communities offer transportation services to the elderly so that they can make it to their medical appointments or exercise classes. Community centers and senior centers offer low-cost nutritious meals. Meals-on-wheels brings prepared meals to your home. Volunteers who visit shut-ins may be available. Local diabetes organizations may offer classes or support groups. To find out what services are available in your area, check your local yellow pages, ask your health-care team, or call the elder care locator at: 1-800-677-1116.

CHAPTER 16

How Sweet It Is: A Look at Sugars and Sweeteners

✑

IN THIS CHAPTER

- Sugar
- Other calorie-containing sweeteners
- Stevia
- Artificial sweeteners
- Recipe conversions between sugar and artificial sweeteners

The use of sugar, sweeteners, and sugar substitutes has often been a topic of hot debate. Until recently, using sugar has been discouraged in diabetic meal planning. Current scientific studies have not supported the necessity of completely abstaining from sugar, and now it's becoming widely accepted that sugar may be used in moderation without causing deterioration in blood sugar control.

Countless studies have investigated the safety profiles of artificial sweeteners. This chapter touches on four artificial sweeteners that received approval by the Food and Drug Administration (FDA).

Misinformation is rampant regarding the safety and acceptability of using both sugar and artificial sweeteners. A fair amount of alarmist propaganda is out there, mixed in with medical facts. Listen with a critical ear. Try to review the scientific studies, not the hearsay. Consider the source of the information. In the end, the decision is up to you.

Sugar

Historically, people with diabetes were advised to completely avoid eating sugar, in hopes that this would control their blood sugar. More recently, it's become clear that strict avoidance of dietary sugar is unnecessary. Studies have shown that when sugar is eaten in reasonable amounts and in the context of a healthful diet, blood sugar control is not jeopardized. Keep in mind that all carbohydrates (except fiber) are digested and then absorbed as sugar into the bloodstream. Blacklisting one form of carbohydrate will not cure diabetes. What's more important is eating a reasonable amount of total carbohydrate. *How much carbohydrate you eat and how it is spaced throughout the day are much more influential on the blood sugar than the specific type of carbohydrate you choose.* Although you may include refined sugar in the diet, it's wise to moderate the amount of sugar that you consume. Sugary foods are often low in nutritional value, high in fat or calories, or all three.

> More recently, it's become clear that strict avoidance of dietary sugar is unnecessary.

There are naturally occurring sugars, as well as added sugars. Fruit and milk both have natural forms of sugar (fructose and lactose, respectively). Naturally occurring sugars and added sugars affect the blood sugar similarly. In other words, if you consume 15 grams of carbohydrate in the form of an apple or 15 grams of carbohydrate in the form of a cookie, the same amount of sugar ends up in the bloodstream. Of course, the fruit is a far more healthful choice. Fruit offers important nutrients, including vitamins, minerals, and fiber. Fruit doesn't have any fat, either. Lightning won't strike you down for eating the occasional cookie, but the diet police (well-intentioned family, friends, and strangers) may swarm around you, scolding that people with diabetes can't eat sugar. Everyone has been so conditioned to believe that sugar is evil that it's been hard to dispel this myth.

Some sugar-sweetened items do tend to raise the blood sugar quickly. For example, it doesn't take long to digest liquids, so the sugar from regular sodas and sugary drinks can enter the bloodstream rapidly. A 12-ounce can of soda (45 grams carbohydrate) is roughly equal to 9 teaspoons of sugar. Fruit juice has almost the same amount of sugar, it's just a different type of sugar. Use caution with both regular soda and fruit juice. You may find that your blood sugar is easier to control if you use diet drinks instead.

> Blacklisting one form of carbohydrate will not cure diabetes. What's more important is eating a reasonable amount of total carbohydrate.

Also, be aware that goopy, frosted goodies can have a large amount of carbohydrate concentrated in a relatively small portion.

Tip: Diet soft drinks do not affect the blood sugar.

Tip: One tablespoon of sugar has about 15 grams of carbohydrate.

Other Calorie-Containing Sweeteners

Honey, maple syrup, pancake syrup, malt syrup, corn syrup, Karo syrup, corn sweeteners, molasses, jelly, jam, and marmalade are all concentrated forms of sweeteners. There's no advantage or disadvantage to using any one of these over another. They'll all affect the blood sugar similarly. They each contribute approximately 15 grams of carbohydrate per tablespoon, which is about the same as white sugar.

Fructose

Fructose is the sugar that occurs naturally in fruits. (Fruit also contains glucose.) Powdered fructose may have some advantage over white sugar because it produces a smaller rise in blood sugar than the same amount of white sugar. Since fructose tastes sweeter than sugar, less can be used. Fructose can be used in baking.

Fructose doesn't require digestion in the intestines. It gets absorbed into the bloodstream as fructose, not glucose. Fructose is then transported to the liver, where it's converted to glucose and stored as glycogen for later use. It's released into the bloodstream as needed.

Studies have shown that when a very large intake of fructose was eaten (20 percent of total calories), the undesirable kind of blood cholesterol (LDL cholesterol) went up. Don't give up fruit if you have high cholesterol, though. Just use moderation in the amount of fructose-sweetened products you use.

Sugar Alcohol

Mannitol, maltitol, lactitol, xylitol, sorbitol, hydrogenated starch hydrolysate, and isomalt are all sugar alcohols. Sugar alcohols don't contain sugar or alcohol, but they are a type of carbohydrate. Sugar alcohols don't impact the blood sugar as much as regular sugars, but they do still eventually produce some glucose in the blood. Since sugar alcohols aren't technically a form of sugar, products sweetened with sugar alcohols can boast that they are "sugar-free." That doesn't necessarily mean the product is "carbohydrate-free" or "low calorie." Most chocolates that are sweetened with sugar alcohols have just as much fat, calories, and total carbohydrate as regular chocolate candies. However, sugar alcohols don't promote tooth decay.

Lightning won't strike you down for eating the occasional cookie, but the diet police (well-intentioned family, friends, and strangers) may swarm around you, scolding that people with diabetes can't eat sugar.

Since sugar alcohols don't raise the blood sugar as much as an equal amount of regular sugar, they shouldn't be used to treat low blood sugar.

Sugar alcohols may have a laxative effect, causing gas, bloating, and diarrhea. Tolerance varies from one individual to the next but is usually related to the amount of sugar alcohol consumed. There are no other safety issues.

Read food labels. The amount of sugar alcohol will be listed under the total grams of carbohydrate. The ingredient list can identify the types of sugar alcohol used.

Stevia

Stevia is a natural sweetening substance made from a South American shrub. It has been used to sweeten foods for many years in other countries. It has not yet received FDA approval to be sold as a sweetener in the United States. To gain FDA approval, safety studies will have to be performed and submitted to the FDA. Stevia is available in some health food stores, where it is sold as a "dietary supplement." It cannot be packaged and labeled as a "sweetener."

Artificial Sweeteners

The FDA has approved the following artificial sweeteners for use in the United States. The acceptable daily intake (ADI) has a built-in 100-fold safety factor. The amounts that people actually consume are well below what has been determined to be safe.

Aspartame is sold under the brand names Equal, NutraSweet, SweetMate, and NatraTaste. The FDA approved aspartame in 1981. It is 180 times sweeter than sugar. If heated at extreme temperatures, aspartame loses its sweetness; therefore, it is not acceptable for use in most cooked or baked goods.

Aspartame is made of two amino acids: phenylalanine and aspartic acid. Amino acids are the natural building blocks of proteins. When aspartame is digested into its amino acid components, the body cannot distinguish whether those amino acids came from aspartame or from dietary proteins like chicken, milk, or eggs.

Small amounts of methanol are produced as a by-product from digesting aspartame. Methanol is a by-product that is also produced from digesting the regular foods that we eat. Natural juices, including fruit juice and tomato juice, produce three to six times more methanol than an equal portion of aspartame-sweetened soft drink.

There has been a lot of finger-pointing in the direction of aspartame, but claims that it is harmful haven't been substantiated. Whether to use aspartame or not is a matter of personal choice.

Patients with a very rare metabolic disease called PKU (phenylketonuria) should not use aspartame because they need to limit all sources of phenylalanine.

Acesulfame K is sold under the brand names Sunett, Swiss Sweet, and Sweet One. Gaining FDA approval in 1988, acesulfame K is 200 times sweeter than sugar. It is heat stable and can be used in baking. No safety concerns have been raised.

Sucralose is sold under the brand name Splenda. The FDA approved Sucralose in 1998. It's actually made out of sugar but has been modified so that it doesn't affect the blood sugar or provide any calories. It's 600 times sweeter than sugar. It's stable at high temperatures and can be used in baked goods. Like the other artificial sweeteners, sucralose doesn't promote tooth decay.

> Studies have shown that when a very large intake of fructose was eaten (20 percent of total calories), the undesirable kind of blood cholesterol (LDL cholesterol) went up.

Saccharin is sold under the brand name Sweet 'N Low. Saccharin has been around since 1879. It's approximately 300 times sweeter than sugar. It's stable when heated, so it can be used in baking. In the 1970s its safety came under question, as some studies showed that rats that were fed large amounts of saccharin developed bladder tumors. Saccharin has been scrutinized and studied over the past several decades and has now been determined to pose no cancer risks to humans. In May 2000, saccharin was removed from the government's list of carcinogens (cancer-causing substances). The label warning that appears on saccharin will likely soon be dropped.

Recipe Conversions Between Sugar and Artificial Sweeteners

- Each individual packet of Equal, NutraSweet, NatraTaste, Sweet One, Splenda, or Sweet 'N Low provides the same sweetness as 2 teaspoons of sugar.

- Tablets of Equal are each as sweet as 1 teaspoon of sugar.

Table 16.1   Conversion Table for Baking and Cooking

Sugar	¼ cup	⅓ cup	½ cup	1 cup
Equal				
—packets	6 packets	8 packets	12 packets	24 packets
—for recipes	1¾ tsp.	2½ tsp.	3½ tsp.	7¼ tsp.
—spoonful	¼ cup	⅓ cup	½ cup	1 cup
NatraTaste				
—packets	6 packets	8 packets	12 packets	24 packets
—bulk	2 tsp.	2½ tsp.	4 tsp.	8 tsp.
Sweet One				
—packets	6 packets	8 packets	12 packets	24 packets
Splenda				
—packets	6 packets	8 packets	12 packets	24 packets
—bulk	¼ cup	⅓ cup	½ cup	1 cup
Sweet 'N Low				
—packets	6 packets	8 packets	12 packets	24 packets
—bulk	2 tsp.	2½ tsp.	4 tsp.	8 tsp.
—liquid	1½ tsp.	2 tsp.	1 tbsp.	2 tbsp.
—brown	1 tsp.	1¼ tsp.	2 tsp.	4 tsp.

Table 16.1 can be used to find the amount of artificial sweetener needed to provide the same amount of sweetening power as sugar. The top row shows the measurement of sugar. The following rows show the amount of artificial sweetener needed to match sugar's sweetness.

Tip: You can use the equivalent amount of artificial sweetener to replace 100 percent of the sugar used to make fruit fillings, custards, beverages, marinades, relishes, and sauces. That's not true with most baked goods. Baked goods attribute their texture and volume to qualities imparted by sugar. If you take all of the sugar out of the recipe and replace it with an artificial sweetener, the baked good may be "no good." Without any sugar in the recipe, the baked item may not brown properly and may not have the proper volume, moistness, or crumb. Try replacing half of the sugar in the recipe with an equivalent amount of artificial sweetener. Or, you can play it safe and use recipes that have been tested by the manufacturer of the artificial sweetener. Obtain recipes online via the Web sites, or call or write to the company.

Web Sites

www.nutrasweet.com

www.natrataste.com

www.sweetone.com

www.splenda.com

www.sweetnlow.com

Phone Numbers

Equal: 1-800-323-5316

NutraSweet: 1-800-234-5859

NatraTaste: 1-800-628-7211

Sweet One: 1-800-544-8610

Splenda: 1-800-777-5363

Sweet 'N Low: 1-800-221-1763

CHAPTER 17

The Lowdown on Low Blood Sugar

∽

IN THIS CHAPTER

- What is hypoglycemia?
- What causes hypoglycemia?
- The body's response to low blood sugar
- Signs and symptoms of hypoglycemia
- Treating hypoglycemia
- Preventing hypoglycemia

The technical term for low blood sugar is *hypoglycemia*. Having diabetes doesn't necessarily mean that you'll have bouts of hypoglycemia. Hypoglycemia does not result directly from the diabetes, but it can result from some of the medicines that are used to treat diabetes. Certain diabetes medications actively lower the blood sugar. If too much medication is taken or not enough food is eaten, then the blood sugar can go too low. The medications most likely to cause low blood sugar are insulin, sulfonylureas, or meglitinides. If you don't take any medications for your diabetes, then you won't be at risk for getting low blood sugar.

What Is Hypoglycemia?

The word *hypo-gly-cemia* literally means "low sugar in the blood." The body is fussy. It doesn't like too much sugar in the blood, but it doesn't like too little sugar in the blood either. If the sugar in the blood (blood glucose) is too low, there's a shortage of fuel available for the body. The brain and other vital organs rely on glucose to operate properly.

A blood sugar value under 70 mg/dl typically indicates hypoglycemia. Small children, the elderly, and individuals with certain medical conditions may be advised by their health care providers to keep their blood sugar levels over 100 mg/dl.

What Causes Hypoglycemia?
Medication-Related Causes of Hypoglycemia

Insulin is the name of the hormone that lowers the blood sugar. Insulin is necessary to move glucose from the bloodstream into the cells where it's needed. The pancreas is the organ in the body that makes insulin. Normally, the pancreas makes insulin as needed, then stops making insulin once the blood sugar reaches the lower normal limit. Stopping the insulin production ensures that the blood sugar doesn't drop too low.

Some people with diabetes require insulin injections. If the pancreas can't produce adequate amounts of insulin or if the insulin produced by the pancreas doesn't lower the blood sugar sufficiently, supplemental insulin may be prescribed. Anyone who injects insulin is potentially at risk for getting low blood sugar. The difference between injected insulin and insulin made in the body is that injected insulin can't be turned off once the blood sugar reaches the lower limits of normal. Low blood sugar can result any time too much insulin is injected.

Insulin isn't the only diabetes medication that can cause hypoglycemia. Some diabetes pills (oral hypoglycemic agents) work by stimulating the pancreas to make more insulin. Sulfonylureas and meglitinides are classes of drugs that can cause hypoglycemia. Many brand names and generic drugs fall into these classes of medications. (See chapter 2 for more information on diabetes medications.) Although some diabetes pills have the potential to cause low blood sugar, other diabetes pills pose very little, or no, risk for hypoglycemia. Be sure to ask your health-care provider whether you take any diabetes medications that could put you at risk for low blood sugar.

> Hypoglycemia does not result directly from the diabetes, but it can result from some of the medicines that are used to treat diabetes.

Take your medications as directed by your health-care provider. The amount and timing of the dose are both important.

Tip: If you forget a dose in the morning, it isn't a good idea to double up on the next dose. To do so could cause significant hypoglycemia.

Food-Related Causes of Hypoglycemia

If you use insulin or any diabetes pills that stimulate the production of insulin, then you must eat your meals on time. The medications prescribed to you assume that carbohydrate will be eaten in a timely manner and in adequate amounts. Low blood sugar can occur if you eat too little carbohydrate, or if you delay or skip meals. Be sure to follow your meal plan and eat the recommended number of meals and snacks.

Drinking alcohol on an empty stomach, drinking alcohol without adequate carbohydrate intake, or drinking excessive amounts of alcohol can all result in problems with hypoglycemia.

Exercise-Induced Hypoglycemia

A regular exercise routine is an important part of diabetes management. Exercise burns glucose as well as body fat. Medications that lower blood sugar can have an even stronger effect if exercise is more vigorous than usual. Unusually strenuous exercise, prolonged exercise, or unplanned exercise may require additional carbohydrate-containing snacks. If you start an exercise program and become more active on a regular basis, check with your doctor about the possibility of decreasing your diabetes medication doses. If you find yourself getting low blood sugar during or after exercise, then you probably need medication adjustments. Eating more food every time you exercise sort of defeats the purpose. Instead of burning body fat, you just burn the snack you ate!

Causes of Hypoglycemia

Too much injected insulin

Too much or too strong a dose of diabetes pills

Improper timing between diabetes medication and meals

Skipped or delayed meals or snacks

Not eating enough carbohydrate

More exercise than usual

Drinking alcohol on an empty stomach

The Body's Response to Low Blood Sugar

When the blood sugar drops below normal limits, the body does its best to compensate. Luckily, the body stores some glucose in the muscles and the liver. The storage form of glucose is called glycogen. Glycogen is just a long chain of glucose molecules connected together. When glucose is needed, the liver can break down its glycogen stores and release glucose into the blood. When the demand warrants it, the liver can even make new glucose. *Gluconeo-genesis* is the term for making sugar in the body. *Gluco-neo-genesis* means "sugar-new-production."

> The body is fussy. It doesn't like too much sugar in the blood, but it doesn't like too little sugar in the blood either.

The liver, and even the kidneys (to some extent), can take the building blocks from proteins (amino acids) and convert them into glucose. (Drinking alcohol inhibits this production of glucose.

When the liver is busy processing alcohol, it cannot make new glucose. That's why alcohol can cause low blood sugar problems.) The body really is amazing. What it won't do to make sure there's enough fuel to keep the brain and other vital organs properly fueled with glucose!

Hormones (chemical messengers in the body) stimulate the production and release of glucose. Hormones that raise the blood sugar include adrenaline (epinephrine), glucagon, cortisol, and growth hormone. Remember that insulin is the hormone that lowers blood sugar. Just about all other hormones can raise the blood sugar.

> Anyone who injects insulin is potentially at risk for getting low blood sugar.

When prescribed correctly and taken correctly, both insulin and diabetes pills can work well at controlling blood sugar levels without causing hypoglycemia. If too much medication is taken (in relation to the food intake and activity level), the body will attempt to raise the blood sugar on its own. If the body's defenses are no match for the amount of medication present, hypoglycemia will result.

Signs and Symptoms of Hypoglycemia

Many symptoms of low blood sugar can be attributed to the release of hormones that are trying to raise the blood sugar. Adrenaline (epinephrine) is one hormone that raises the blood sugar. Adrenaline is also a hormone released in stressful situations. If you were walking through the jungle and a lion crossed your path, your heart would pound; you'd breathe hard and tremble. All of those symptoms result from the release of adrenaline. In the jungle, adrenaline causes the release of sugar so that you have sufficient fuel for "fight or flight." In the case of hypoglycemia, adrenaline helps to release sugar to rescue you from low blood sugar.

If blood sugar levels drop very low, symptoms may include confusion and lack of coordination because the brain has insufficient amounts of glucose to direct normal bodily functions (see table 17.1).

Table 17.1   Signs and Symptoms of Hypoglycemia

Mild	Moderate to Severe
hunger	headache
trembling	slow thinking
rapid heartbeat	lack of coordination
increased pulse	trouble concentrating
sweating	blurred vision
heavy breathing	anger
tingling	dizziness
nausea	slurred speech
weakness	seizure
nightmares	coma

It isn't possible to predict an absolute blood sugar value that will cause specific symptoms of hypoglycemia. Some individuals feel minimal symptoms for mildly reduced blood sugar levels, while other individuals feel very symptomatic. Keep in mind that you can't predict what your blood sugar is by the way that you feel. It's possible to feel like you have low blood sugar, when in fact your blood sugar level might be perfectly normal or even elevated. It's important to check your blood sugar with your blood sugar monitor (whenever possible) before treating for hypoglycemia.

If you've been running high blood sugar values for some time, your body gets used to those blood sugar levels. (That doesn't mean it's healthy! It just means you feel normal even though your blood sugar is too high.) If you bring your blood sugar levels into a more normal range, your body may register that the blood sugar level is lower than usual and it may sound a false alarm. You can get the *symptoms* of low blood sugar just because your sugar is lower than you're used to. That's a false alarm. You don't need to eat anything if indeed your blood sugar is in the normal range. (Remember that hypoglycemia is typically defined as below 70 mg/dl.) As your blood sugar control improves from day to day, your body will recalibrate and you'll stop having these false alarms.

Treating Hypoglycemia

Most hypoglycemic episodes can be treated simply by eating some carbohydrates. It's best if the carbohydrate source is low in fat and low in protein. Both fat and protein can slow down digestion. If your blood sugar is low, you should eat something that will digest quickly to provide the needed glucose. If the blood sugar is below 70 mg/dl, eat 15 grams of carbohydrate, wait 15 minutes, and test the blood sugar again to ensure that the blood sugar has risen sufficiently.

The rule of 15

Treat low blood sugar with 15 grams of carbohydrate.

Wait 15 minutes.

If the blood sugar has not risen 30 to 50 points, repeat procedure.

You might notice that the *symptoms* of hypoglycemia persist for 15–20 minutes even after you eat the carbohydrate. It takes time for the shakiness and other symptoms to subside. Remember that many symptoms of low blood sugar can be attributed to the release of hormones. Once hormones are released in response to hypoglycemia, it takes time for those hormones to settle down. If you were to continue eating until you felt better, you might end up eating too much. The result could be that your blood sugar then goes too

> Low blood sugar can occur if you eat too little carbohydrate, or if you delay or skip meals.

high. It can turn into a roller coaster. Swinging sugars can be very frustrating. Don't over-treat hypoglycemia.

If your meter shows a low reading but you question the accuracy of the reading, retest your blood sugar. Keep in mind that insufficient blood on a test strip could give a false reading on your blood sugar meter. Make sure that your blood sugar testing technique is correct.

> If you find yourself getting low blood sugar during or after exercise, then you probably need medication adjustments.

Low blood sugar needs to be treated even if you don't feel any symptoms. If the blood sugar is below 70 mg/dl, treat it.

Very low blood sugar levels may require more than 15 grams of carbohydrate to correct them. When choosing the amount of carbohydrate to eat, consider your blood sugar value, the amount of medication in your system, the amount and timing of your last meal, and the effects of any recent exercise.

Appropriate carbohydrate choices used to treat hypoglycemia include glucose tablets, fruit juice, regular soda, hard candies, fruit, or any other fat-free sugar source. Read labels on hard candies for portions equal to 15 grams of carbohydrate.

Don't use donuts, ice cream, candy bars, pie, or cookies. Those items all contain too much fat, which will slow down the digestion and availability of the carbohydrate.

The following list contains appropriate carbohydrate choices to use to treat hypoglycemia. Each portion listed contains about 15 grams of carbohydrate.

Carbohydrate Sources for Treating Hypoglycemia

3–4 glucose tablets

½ cup orange, apple, or pineapple juice

⅓ cup prune, grape, or cranberry juice

½ cup regular soda (not diet)

1 small apple, orange, pear, peach, or banana

2 tablespoons of raisins

1 cup nonfat milk

1 tablespoon of sugar, honey, or syrup (can mix in water if desired)

Once you've treated your low blood sugar reaction and tested your blood sugar to confirm that it's back in the normal range, stop and consider when your next meal or snack will be. If the next meal or snack is over an hour away, then you should probably have a small snack to hold you over. Having a snack with some carbohydrate plus some protein can help prevent a repeated hypoglycemic episode.

If you take any medication that can cause hypoglycemia, you should always carry an appropriate source of carbohydrate with you in case you need it. Keep something nonperishable in the car's glove box, your purse, your desk at work, and your pocket. It's also a good idea to wear some form of identification that states that you have diabetes. Medical alert bracelets, clips for watches, or necklaces are available.

> If blood sugar levels drop very low, symptoms may include confusion and lack of coordination because the brain has insufficient amounts of glucose to direct normal bodily functions.

Preventing Hypoglycemia

It's important to follow up with your health-care provider regularly. You may be evaluated for new types of medications, or your current medication doses may need to be adjusted. Medication doses often need to be reduced once you start an exercise program, improve your food choices, or lose some weight. Monitor your blood sugar, write down the results, and review the values with your health-care provider.

Preventing Hypoglycemia

- See your health-care provider regularly.
- Follow medication-dosing recommendations.

- Monitor your blood sugar regularly.
- Eat all scheduled meals and snacks *on time*.
- Don't skip meals.
- Eat consistent amounts of carbohydrate.
- Don't drink alcohol on an empty stomach (include carbohydrate in the meal).
- If you choose to drink alcohol, use moderate amounts (not more than 1–2 drinks).
- Eat extra carbohydrate snacks for unplanned, prolonged, or strenuous exercise.
- Carry a source of carbohydrate with you in case of hypoglycemia.

CHAPTER 18

Fiber Facts

❧

IN THIS CHAPTER

- Soluble fiber
- Insoluble fiber
- Benefits and sources of fiber
- Fiber content of select foods

Fiber comes from plant foods. Animal products such as meats and dairy products do not contribute fiber. Fiber is the part of the plant food that is not digestible. It's actually a type of carbohydrate, but our digestive enzymes can't break it down into its glucose units, so it doesn't contribute to the blood sugar. By the way, since fiber doesn't get digested, it doesn't contribute any calories.

There are two main types of fiber: soluble and insoluble. Fiber that absorbs water is considered soluble, while fiber that doesn't absorb water is called insoluble. Recommended intake for fiber is 20–35 grams per day from a combination of foods. To help ensure an adequate intake of fiber, it's suggested that we eat at least five portions per day from a combination of fruits and vegetables, as well as at least six servings from the grains and starch group. Try to include more whole grains and less refined grain products.

Food labels provide information on fiber content. For foods that do not have food labels, refer to the list provided at the end of this chapter.

Soluble Fiber

Soluble fiber absorbs water. Oatmeal gets gooey because the soluble fiber holds water. The same goes for split peas and dried beans. This quality provides a benefit that may help lower your blood cholesterol. Soluble fiber forms a gel, and, as the gel moves through the intestines, it absorbs bile. (Bile is a digestive juice that is made by the liver.) Bile normally is reused over and over again, but when it gets trapped in the soluble fiber gel it's eliminated with the rest of the digestive waste products (in other words it's flushed down the toilet). The liver will need to make more bile to replace what was lost. The liver uses cholesterol out of the bloodstream to make bile. And there you have it: Using cholesterol out of your bloodstream to make new bile means that your blood cholesterol level is lowered. Emphasize an intake of soluble fiber to appreciate its cholesterol-lowering effect.

> To help ensure an adequate intake of fiber, it's suggested that we eat at least five portions per day from a combination of fruits and vegetables, as well as at least six servings from the grains and starch group.

Soluble fiber may play a factor in weight control. By producing a feeling of fullness, a diet rich in soluble fiber may result in eating smaller quantities of food. Soluble fiber also plays a role in keeping your intestines and colon healthy.

Insoluble Fiber

Insoluble fiber doesn't absorb water. For example, you could mix bran flakes into a glass of water and come back a day later and the fiber would still be floating on the top. Insoluble fiber does not form a gel, so it doesn't help to lower blood cholesterol levels. It does, however, have other important health benefits. Insoluble fiber moves through the intestines intact and provides bulk. It promotes bowel regularity by preventing constipation and helps to keep the colon and intestines healthy. (See table 18.1 for the health benefits of soluble and insoluble fiber.)

Fiber Content of Select Foods

Table 18.2 can be used to count grams of fiber. If you don't care to count the grams of fiber you eat, use the table to compare foods and

Table 18.1   Fiber: Benefits and Best Sources

Soluble	Insoluble
Benefits	
Helps lower blood cholesterol	Colon health
May help with weight control	Prevents constipation
Colon health	
Sources	
Legumes/dried beans and peas	Whole wheat
Fruits. Especially: apples, apricots, mangos, peaches, strawberries, oranges, papaya	Bran flakes
	Whole grains
Vegetables. Especially: carrots, Brussels sprouts, sweet potatoes, asparagus, broccoli, and turnips	Vegetables—especially their skins
	Fruits—especially their skins
Oat bran, oatmeal, barley	Legumes/dried beans and peas
Fiber supplements that contain psyllium	Popcorn

choose the higher-fiber options. Meats, eggs, and dairy products are not included in the table because they don't have any fiber.

The fiber content is listed in grams. Note: The serving sizes for grains, legumes and vegetables are all measured *after* the foods are cooked.

Table 18.2

Food Item	Serving Size	Total Fiber	Soluble Fiber	Insoluble Fiber
Grains:				
white pasta	½ cup	0.9	0.4	0.5
wheat pasta	½ cup	2.7	0.6	2.1
white rice	⅓ cup	0.5	trace	0.5
wild rice	⅓ cup	0.4	0.1	0.3
Other:				
popcorn	3 cups	2.0	0.1	1.9
wheat bran	3 tablespoons	4.6	0.4	4.2
wheat germ	3 tablespoons	3.9	0.7	3.2
Breads and Crackers:				
white bread	1 slice	0.6	0.3	0.3
wheat bread	1 slice	1.5	0.3	1.2
rye bread	1 slice	1.8	0.8	1.0
raisin bread	1 slice	1.2	0.3	0.9
burger bun	½ bun	0.7	0.2	0.5
English muffin	½	0.8	0.2	0.6
corn tortilla	1 small	1.4	0.2	1.2
flour tortilla	1 small	0.7	0.3	0.4
toaster waffle	1	0.7	0.3	0.4
pretzels	¾ ounce	0.8	0.2	0.6
saltine crackers	6	0.5	0.3	0.2
matzo	1	1.0	0.5	0.5
Cereals:				
All Bran	⅓ cup	8.6	1.4	7.2
Cheerios	1¼ cups	2.5	1.2	1.3

Table 18.2   (continued)

Food Item	Serving Size	Total Fiber	Soluble Fiber	Insoluble Fiber
Cereals (continued):				
Corn Flakes	1 cup	0.5	0.1	0.4
Fiber One	½ cup	11.9	0.8	11.1
40% Bran Flakes	⅔ cup	4.3	0.4	3.9
Grapenuts	¼ cup	2.8	0.8	2.0
Oat Bran Flakes	½ cup	2.1	0.8	0.3
Product 19	1 cup	1.2	0.3	0.9
Puffed Wheat	1 cup	1.0	0.5	0.5
Raisin Bran	¾ cup	5.3	0.9	4.4
Rice Krispies	1 cup	0.3	0.1	0.2
Shredded Wheat	⅔ cup	3.5	0.5	3.5
Special K	1 cup	0.9	0.2	0.7
Wheaties	⅔ cup	2.3	0.7	1.6
Fruits:				
apple	1 small	2.8	1.0	1.8
applesauce	½ cup	2.0	0.7	1.3
apricots	4 fresh	3.5	1.8	1.7
banana	½ small	1.1	0.3	0.8
blueberries	¾ cup	1.4	0.3	1.1
cantaloupe	1 cup	1.1	0.3	0.8
cherries	12 fresh	1.3	0.6	0.7
dates	2½	0.9	0.3	0.6
figs	1½ dried	2.3	1.1	1.2
grapefruit	½	1.6	1.1	0.5
grapes	15	0.6	0.3	0.3
honeydew	1 cup	0.9	0.3	0.6
kiwi	1 large	1.7	0.7	1.0
mango	½ small	2.9	1.7	1.2
nectarine	1 small	1.8	0.8	1.0
orange	1 small	2.9	1.8	1.1

Table 18.2   (continued)

Food Item	Serving Size	Total Fiber	Soluble Fiber	Insoluble Fiber
Fruits (continued):				
peach	1 medium	2.0	1.0	1.0
pear	1 small	2.9	1.1	1.8
pineapple	¾ cup fresh	1.4	0.1	1.3
plums	2 medium	2.4	1.1	1.3
prunes	3	1.7	1.0	0.7
raisins	2 tablespoons	0.4	0.2	0.2
raspberries	1 cup	3.3	0.9	2.4
strawberries	1¼ cups	2.8	1.1	1.7
watermelon	1¼ cups	0.6	0.4	0.2
Vegetables:				
asparagus	½ cup	2.8	1.7	1.1
beets	½ cup	1.8	0.8	1.0
broccoli	½ cup	2.4	1.2	1.2
brussels sprouts	½ cup	3.8	2.0	1.8
cabbage, red	½ cup	2.6	1.1	1.5
carrots	½ cup	2.0	1.1	0.9
cauliflower	½ cup	1.0	0.4	0.6
corn	½ cup	1.6	0.2	1.4
green beans	½ cup	2.8	1.1	1.7
kale	½ cup	2.5	0.7	1.8
lettuce	1 cup	0.5	0.1	0.4
okra	½ cup	4.1	1.0	3.1
peas, frozen	½ cup	4.3	1.3	3.0
sweet potato	⅓ cup	2.7	1.2	1.5
snow peas	½ cup	1.4	0.6	0.8
spinach	½ cup	1.6	0.5	1.1
tomato sauce	⅓ cup	1.1	0.5	0.6
turnip	½ cup	4.8	1.7	3.1
zucchini	½ cup	1.2	0.5	0.7

Table 18.2   (continued)

Food Item	Serving Size	Total Fiber	Soluble Fiber	Insoluble Fiber
Legumes:				
black beans	½ cup	6.1	2.4	3.7
black-eyed peas	½ cup	4.7	0.5	4.2
broad beans	½ cup	5.1	1.0	4.1
butter beans	½ cup	6.9	2.7	4.2
chick peas	½ cup	4.3	1.3	3.0
kidney beans	½ cup	6.9	2.8	4.1
lentils	½ cup	5.2	0.6	4.6
lima beans	½ cup	4.3	1.1	3.2
navy beans	½ cup	6.5	2.2	4.3
pinto beans	½ cup	5.9	1.9	4.0
split peas	½ cup	3.1	1.1	2.0
Nuts and Seeds:				
almonds	6 nuts	0.6	0.1	0.5
hazelnuts	1 tablespoon	0.5	0.2	0.3
peanut butter	1 tablespoon	1.0	0.3	0.7
peanuts	10	0.6	0.2	0.4
sesame seeds	1 tablespoon	0.8	0.2	0.6
sunflower seeds	1 tablespoon	0.5	0.2	0.3
walnuts	2 whole	0.3	0.1	0.2

CHAPTER 19

Alcohol Advice

⌘

IN THIS CHAPTER

- Alcohol metabolism
- Alcohol's effect on the triglycerides (blood fats)
- Alcohol's effect on the liver
- Alcohol's effect on the blood sugar
- Alcohol's effect on weight
- Liquor: A look at calories and carbs
- General warnings

I 'll jump to the punch line on this one: It's okay to include a moderate amount of alcohol if your diabetes is well controlled and you don't have any other reasons that you should abstain. If in doubt, check with your health-care provider for clearance. Some medical conditions require complete abstinence, and alcohol can react dangerously with certain medications. Moderation means one to two drinks per day. The usual recommendation is no more than one drink per day for the smaller body size (or women) and not more than two drinks per day for the larger person (or men). One "drink" is equal to one 12-ounce beer, one 5-ounce glass of wine, or 1½ ounces of distilled alcohol (a "shot" of hard liquor). Each of those servings provides about the same amount of alcohol.

Note: To figure out how much pure alcohol is in the beverage, divide the "proof" in half. For example, something that is 80 proof is 40 percent pure ethanol alcohol.

Alcohol itself doesn't raise your blood sugar. Sure, some alcoholic beverages have added sugars and sweet mixers, which definitely do contribute to the blood glucose, but a shot of distilled spirits doesn't turn into sugar in the blood. In fact, in some instances, alcohol can actually cause a low blood sugar reaction (hypoglycemia).

Alcohol Metabolism

Metabolism is the term that describes how something is broken down in the body and what happens to the by-products. Alcohol is absorbed into the bloodstream through the stomach and the intestines. It's absorbed very quickly, within minutes. You know what I mean if you've ever had a drink on an empty stomach. Alcohol then journeys to the liver, where it is dismantled, or broken down. The end products are fatty acids (fats) which can be used for fuel, or stored in the body for later use.

> Alcohol is metabolized similarly to fat, which means it can affect your triglycerides (blood fats), as well as your weight.

The metabolism of alcohol results in many metabolic disturbances. Alcohol gets preferential treatment because the body sees it as a toxic substance, which must be dismantled. What it boils down to is that the liver becomes busy breaking down the alcohol, resulting in other important bodily processes being put on hold.

Alcohol's Effect on the Triglycerides (Blood Fats)

Metabolism of alcohol can result in an overproduction of triglycerides, which are the fats that circulate in the blood. High triglycerides can contribute to heart disease, and extremely high triglycerides can cause pancreatitis (inflammation and injury to the pancreas). If you have a history of high triglycerides, you should avoid alcohol completely.

Alcohol's Effect on the Liver

Heavy drinking can cause fat to accumulate in the liver. In time, liver cells die and are replaced with scar tissue. This is known as fibrosis, which can eventually lead to a serious and life threatening liver disease called cirrhosis.

Alcohol's Effect on the Blood Sugar

The liver has many functions, one of which is to help regulate blood sugar. If the blood sugar level falls too low, it's the liver's job to release sugar and raise the blood sugar to a safe level. The liver can release sugar that it had stored previously or can make brand-new glucose in a process called gluconeogenesis (gluco-neo-genesis: *gluco* means "glucose," *neo* means "new," and *genesis* means "to make, or create").

As already stated, alcohol is metabolized in the liver. Here's the clincher: When the liver is breaking down alcohol, it can't make new glucose in response to low blood sugar. (It takes about 1–1½ hours to metabolize one drink.) So, if you take insulin or any diabetes pills that can cause low blood sugar, alcohol poses a special risk to you. If you get low blood sugar from your medicine and your liver can't adequately raise your blood sugar levels because you've ingested alcohol, your blood sugar can end up going lower, and lower, and lower. Let's take it a step further. If you've had a drink or two, you may not feel the symptoms of low blood sugar, so you may not realize that you need to eat some carbohydrates. If your blood sugar drops severely, you may be stumbling instead of walking. And guess what? Everyone thinks that you've just had too much to drink and may not realize that you need help. It's a treacherous slope!

Alcohol-induced hypoglycemia is preventable. Some folks choose not to drink, and then they're not at risk. If you choose to drink, drink safely and responsibly. Here are a few tips:

- *Use moderation:* limit yourself to no more than one to two drinks.

- *Don't drink on an empty stomach!* Make sure that you eat carbohydrates. If carbohydrates are digesting and turning into glucose, you're less likely to get low blood sugar in the first place. (Various mixed drinks contain carbohydrate, which may offer some protection against hypoglycemia, but it's still recommended *not* to drink on an empty stomach.)

- *Monitor your blood sugar!* Yes, you need to carry your blood sugar monitor with you. If you're at a nightclub, ask the bartender if you can leave your meter behind the bar while you dance. Your meter won't do you any good if it's left in your car.

- *Don't drink after heavy exercise.* Strenuous or long-duration exercise can increase your risk for low blood sugar. Exercise-induced hypoglycemia can occur hours after the exercise.

- *Carry carbohydrates with you that can be used to treat low blood sugar.* Carry hard candies, jelly beans, fruit, juice, or glucose tablets with you in case you get low blood sugar. See chapter 17 for more tips on treating low blood sugar.

- *Wear medical alert identification.* The symptoms of low blood sugar may mimic intoxication. Identification can assist you in getting the care that you need.

Alcohol's Effect on Weight

If you're counting calories, alcohol adds up, and it adds up fast. Only fat is a more concentrated source of calories. Alcohol has 7 calories per gram. (Fat has 9 calories per gram, and both carbohydrate and protein have 4 calories per gram.) The calories in alcohol are referred to as "empty calories," meaning that they don't offer any significant vitamins or minerals. The mixers used in cocktails can be an additional source of calories and carbohydrate. If you're counting calories, you can use diet sodas, diet tonic, club soda, or water as mixers.

> If you get low blood sugar from your medicine and your liver can't adequately raise your blood sugar levels, your blood sugar can end up going lower, and lower, and lower.

Good news for you chefs: If you use alcohol in cooking, the alcohol evaporates, leaving just the flavor and not the calories.

Liquor: A Look at Calories and Carbs

Table 19.1 provides information on serving size, calories, and carbohydrate content of various alcoholic beverages. The exchange system equivalents are provided to help you account for the calories. For example, a beer is counted as one starch exchange and one fat exchange. That's because beer has some carbohydrate from the barley, malt, and hops, which counts as a starch exchange. The alcohol in beer is counted as a fat exchange. (Alcohol is not a fat, but since it's

> If you take insulin or any diabetes pills that can cause low blood sugar, alcohol poses a special risk to you.

metabolized similarly to fat, it's counted as a fat exchange.) Surprisingly, wine is very low in carbohydrate (with the exception of sweet dessert wines). The grape juice that wine is made from has been converted to alcohol in the fermentation process.

Liqueurs and mixed drinks vary in calories and carbohydrate content, depending on the beverage and the portion size. For example, a coffee-flavored liqueur can have as much as 175 calories and 25 grams of carbohydrate in just a 1½-ounce portion! A piña colada has about 290 calories and 45 grams of carbohydrate in a 5-ounce portion! Liqueurs and mixed drinks are too numerous to include here.

General Warnings

- *Never* drink before driving.
- *Never* drink if you are pregnant.
- Don't give in to social pressures to drink.

Table 19.1   Liquor: A Look at Calories and Carbs

Beverage	Serving Size	Calories	Carbohydrate	Food Exchange
Beer	12 ounces	150	13	1 starch, 1½ fat
Light Beer	12 ounces	110	7	2 fats
Red Wine	5 ounces	100	2	2 fats
Rose Wine	5 ounces	100	2	2 fats
White Wine	5 ounces	100	1	2 fats
Dessert Wine	2 ounces	90	7	2 fats
Gin	1½ ounces	110	0	2½ fats
Rum	1½ ounces	97	0	2 fats
Vodka	1½ ounces	97	0	2 fats
Whiskey	1½ ounces	105	0	2½ fats

CHAPTER 20

Alternative Therapies

᭤

IN THIS CHAPTER

- Plants and herbs that claim to treat diabetes
- Chromium, magnesium, and vanadium
- Antioxidants: vitamin C, vitamin E, beta-carotene, and selenium

Wouldn't it be great if you could take a magic pill that improved your diabetes or, better yet, cured your diabetes, without causing any harmful side effects? What if this pill was something totally natural? Would you tell your doctor that you were taking the natural product in addition to your prescription drugs? Would you stop taking the medication that your doctor had previously prescribed?

Natural products, herbal remedies, and dietary supplements promising to treat diabetes are being promoted via the Internet, health food stores, grocery stores, mail flyers, magazines, and through some drugstores. Whether the claims are true or not, it's estimated that one out of every three Americans have tried alternative therapies to treat their ailments. Natural remedies are big business. Manufacturers of the products are raking in money. The questions remain, Do the products work, and are there any risks?

Let's start by stating that no known cure for diabetes exists at this time. You can't take a pill or a potion and forget about your diabetes.

Lifestyle modifications such as a healthful diet and regular exercise will always be the foundation for treating diabetes effectively. Many prescription drugs are available to treat diabetes. But even taking a prescription drug for your diabetes doesn't mean that you can ignore the importance of taking care of yourself and of leading a healthful lifestyle.

> Natural remedies are big business. Manufacturers of the products are raking in money. The questions remain, Do the products work, and are there any risks?

Relatively few well-conducted studies have focused on the use of alternative therapies, such as herbs, to treat diabetes. In most instances, alternative therapies have not been thoroughly investigated for safety, and there is limited, if any, evidence that these products will work. The FDA's regulation of these products entails removing products only *after* they are shown to be harmful. The product health claims are not closely regulated, and quality and purity of the products are not regulated. Manufacturers may voluntarily abide by the Good Manufacturing Practice (GMP) standards; however, many do not meet these standards. In contrast, prescription drugs have to prove that they're effective and safe. Before a drug is made available to the public, clinical trials must be conducted. These trials must adhere to strict scientific experimental methods. Results are published in reputable medical journals and scrutinized by the scientific community. No similar standards exist for regulating herbal and natural treatments for diabetes. That leaves you, the consumer, vulnerable to false claims and even contaminated products. Before you part with your money, it's important to be critical in your review of alternative therapies. Be wary of products that claim to cure diabetes or eliminate the need for traditional treatments. If those claims were true, we wouldn't have millions of Americans who still have diabetes.

But if it's natural, you might ask, what's the harm of trying it? Many people think that if something is "natural," it can pose no serious risk. Natural products and herbal remedies are not always free from side effects. Many of our prescription drugs are derived from plants. Likewise, herbal and natural remedies may contain potent chemical compounds that have "drug-like" activity. Natural products may have side effects, have toxicity risks, or interact dangerously with other medications that you take. It's important to tell your health-care provider about all the therapies you use, including natural remedies, herbs, prescribed medications, and over-the-counter medications. And if you do use alternative therapies, don't take more than the recommended dose. More is not necessarily better!

Although some herbs and plants do appear to show potential in treating diabetes, these alternative therapies need further investigation to ensure safety and to determine appropriate dosing. At this time, I don't actively promote the use of unregulated products. Quality assurance measures aren't consistent. The products can vary from one manufacturer to the next. Or the products might contain ingredients or contaminants that could be harmful to the consumer. A recent news release from the California Department of Health Services warned consumers that several brands of Chinese herbs that claimed to lower blood sugar were actually found to contain potent prescription drugs in mixture with the herbs. The product labels did not inform consumers of the presence of the drugs. The products were investigated after a person with diabetes suffered serious low blood sugar reactions from taking the herbal supplement.

If you do decide to try an herbal supplement, discuss it with your health-care provider. It's important that your health-care provider be aware of your treatment results to ensure that your diabetes is satisfactorily controlled. A pharmacist can advise you on interactions the herbal preparation could have with other medications that you take.

Let's start by stating that no known cure for diabetes exists at this time. You can't take a pill or a potion and forget about your diabetes.

Make sure that the product package lists all the ingredients and provides the lot number, manufacturer's name, and an expiration date. Stop taking the product if you experience any negative side effects. If you don't see improvement in a couple of months, you probably are wasting your money. Plenty of products out there offer no benefit whatsoever.

Caution: Pregnant and lactating women, as well as children, should not experiment with any unproved alternative therapies.

Besides their increasing interest in natural remedies, many people have questions regarding vitamin and mineral supplementation. Vitamins and minerals have important roles in health and in healing. But does having diabetes increase your need for certain vitamins or minerals? Generally speaking, the answer is no. A well-planned and balanced diet can provide all of the vitamins and minerals you need. If you choose to take a multivitamin and mineral supplement, choose one that supplies 100 percent of the RDA.

Tip: Generic brands work just as well as the more expensive name brand vitamins.

In addition to reviewing several herbs used for treating diabetes, this chapter will address a few key vitamins and minerals that have received attention in the press.

> Although some herbs and plants do appear to show potential in treating diabetes, these alternative therapies need further investigation to ensure safety and to determine appropriate dosing.

Plants and Herbs That Claim to Treat Diabetes

More than 400 herbal products or plants have been said to lower the blood sugar. The following plants and herbs are among those that are claimed to treat diabetes. These select few have received the most attention. Because of lack of standardization and regulation of these products, dose recommendations will not be made here. Large clinical trials are needed for us to better understand which, if any, of these products may be useful in the future. Studies are also needed to prove safety and determine appropriate dosages.

Bitter Melon

Small, uncontrolled trials have shown that bitter melon does have some blood sugar–lowering effect. Side effects that need to be investigated further include the risk of severe low blood sugar and the risk of toxicity to the liver.

Fenugreek

Fenugreek seeds have been shown to lower blood sugar, but it's not clear what the standard dose should be. Possible side effects include gas, diarrhea, and upset stomach.

Ginseng

Ginseng has been shown to lower blood sugar. The compound responsible for lowering the blood sugar has not been isolated. Dosing standards have not been established. Possible side effects include nausea, headache, dizziness, sleeplessness, and nervousness.

Guar Gum

This is actually a form of soluble fiber. It may lower the blood sugar somewhat, but because it doesn't taste good, its use isn't widely accepted. Side effects include intestinal discomfort.

Gymnema Sylvestre

The use of this herb dates back to the 6th century B.C. Presumably, it enhances the action of the body's insulin, which in turn lowers the blood sugar. A perplexing side effect is that it alters the ability to taste bitter and sweet flavors. Long-term side effects and toxicity risks are not known.

Chromium, Magnesium, and Vanadium

When addressing blood sugar management, three dietary supplements seem to receive the most attention. Foremost is chromium. Also sharing the spotlight are magnesium and vanadium.

Chromium

What is it?
Chromium is a trace element.

DIETARY REFERENCE INTAKES

Recommended Dietary Allowance (RDA): The average daily dietary intake level that's sufficient to meet the nutrient requirement of nearly all healthy individuals.

Adequate Intake (AI): A recommended intake that's assumed to be adequate for healthy individuals. This is used when RDAs cannot be determined.

Tolerable Upper Intake Level (UL): The highest level of daily nutrient intake that's likely to pose no adverse risks for most people.

What does it do?

Small amounts of chromium are needed for normal metabolism. Chromium is used to make a substance called glucose tolerance factor, which helps the body's insulin work better.

Chromium Requirements

To date, there's not enough evidence regarding chromium for the policy makers to determine recommended dietary allowances (RDAs). The adult daily intake that has been deemed "adequate" by the National Research Council is as follows:

Adequate Intake (AI) for Chromium (in micrograms)

Women aged 19–50 years:	25
Women aged 51 years or older:	20
Pregnant women aged 19–50:	30
Lactating women aged 19–50:	45
Men aged 19–50 years:	35
Men aged 51 years or older:	30

Who may be deficient in chromium?

- People with poor diets or who are otherwise malnourished

- Chronic dieters who consume less than 1,200 calories per day

- Elderly individuals with poor appetites or poor intake

- Individuals who are on long-term intravenous feedings

Do chromium supplements lower the blood sugar?

If a person has a medically documented chromium deficiency, then supplementation may help to improve the blood sugar. If a person does not have a chromium deficiency, then supplementation would probably not improve the blood sugar. It's recommended that chromium be obtained by eating a healthful, balanced diet. If you do choose to supplement chromium, make sure to read the packaging on the supplement bottle. Chromium supplements often contain other ingredients that may have detrimental side effects.

Tip: People who are well nourished don't tend to be deficient in chromium so it's unlikely that they would benefit from supplementation. Most people with diabetes are not chromium deficient.

What foods contain chromium?

Bran

Brewer's yeast

Cereals

Cheese

Chicken

Liver

Meat

Oysters

Peanuts and peanut butter

Potatoes eaten with the skins on

Wheat germ

Magnesium

What is it?
Magnesium is a mineral.

What does it do?
Magnesium is needed for strong bones and normal muscle and nerve function. Many chemical reactions that take place in the body require magnesium. Magnesium is present in every cell in the body. Magnesium may play a role in the activity of insulin. It has been noted that people who are deficient in magnesium are prone to insulin resistance, which results in elevated blood sugar levels.

Magnesium Requirements

Recommended Dietary Allowance (RDA) for Magnesium (in Milligrams)

Women aged 19–30 years:	310
Women aged 31 years or older:	320
Pregnant women aged 19–30:	350
Pregnant women aged 31–50:	360
Lactating women aged 19–30:	310
Lactating women aged 31–50:	320
Men aged 19–30 years:	400
Men aged 31 years or older:	420

Who may be deficient in magnesium?
It's very difficult to measure magnesium status. Deficiency related to diet is very rare. Magnesium deficiency can occur from the following situations:

- Chronic diarrhea or diseases of the intestinal tract can limit magnesium absorption or increase magnesium depletion.
- Chronic vomiting can cause magnesium deficiency.
- High blood sugar levels associated with poorly controlled diabetes can increase the amount of magnesium lost in the urine.

- Alcoholism can contribute to magnesium deficiency.

- Certain diuretics and various other medications can increase the loss of magnesium in the urine.

Do magnesium supplements lower the blood sugar?

If a person has a medically documented magnesium deficiency, then supplementation may help to improve blood sugar control. If a person does not have a magnesium deficiency, then supplementation would probably not improve the blood sugar. Rather than supplement, it's recommended that magnesium be obtained by eating a healthful, balanced diet.

> Although eating fruits and vegetables has been shown to have health benefits, isolating individual carotenoids and taking them in pill form has not always shown clear-cut health benefits.

What foods contain magnesium?

Avocado

Bananas

Bran

Green vegetables

Kiwi fruit

Legumes (dried beans, split peas, and lentils)

Nuts

Potatoes with the skin on

Seeds

Shrimp

Wheat germ

Whole grains

Vanadium

What is it?

Vanadium is a trace element.

What does it do?

More studies are needed to determine the biological function of vanadium. Vanadium may affect blood sugar, but if so and how are not yet clear.

> A very large intake of dietary carotenoids can produce a yellowing of the skin, as avid drinkers of carrot juice can attest!

Vanadium Requirements

Tolerable Upper Intake Level (UL) for elemental vanadium (in milligrams)—All adults: 1.8

RDAs have not been set because the importance of vanadium in the diet isn't yet clear. Instead, nutrition policy makers have set an upper limit and suggest that adults not routinely exceed 1.8 milligrams of elemental vanadium per day. Safe upper limits haven't been established for children or pregnant or lactating women. It's recommended that those groups of people obtain vanadium through diet alone and not supplements.

Who may be deficient in vanadium?

Vanadium deficiency has not been reported.

Do vanadium supplements lower the blood sugar?

Studies are lacking. The role of vanadium is still uncertain. Vanadium supplementation isn't a recognized treatment for diabetes at this time, and vanadium supplements should be used with caution, due to potential side effects.

What foods contain vanadium?

Black pepper

Dill seeds

Grains

Meat, fish, and poultry

Mushrooms

Parsley

Shellfish

Whole grains

Antioxidants

Antioxidants have received a lot of attention in recent years, in relation to wellness and disease prevention. Studies relating antioxidants to diabetes or the potential complications from diabetes are lacking.

Several vitamins and minerals are classified as antioxidants. An antioxidant is a substance that reduces cellular damage. It has been proposed that antioxidants play a role in disease prevention. Our bodies produce some antioxidants naturally. Certain foods are also good sources of antioxidants. It's well accepted that eating foods rich in antioxidants is a healthful thing to do. The jury is split on whether or not to use vitamin supplements to further boost antioxidant intake. Some studies show benefit from supplementing with antioxidant vitamins, while other studies aren't so conclusive.

Oxidation is a process by which damage occurs as a result of contact with oxygen. Oxidation of iron results in rust, as illustrated by a nail that's exposed to air. Food spoils because of exposure to oxygen in the air. Even though oxygen is essential to humans, we aren't exempt from oxidative damage. We won't rust or spoil; the damage is more discreet. Oxidation leads to the formation of "free radicals." Free radicals form from normal cellular processes. Environmental hazards can increase free radical production. Exposure to the sun's damaging rays, car exhaust, ozone, cigarette smoke, drugs, poisons, and pesticides can all amplify free radical production. (It's not enough to take care of ourselves; we must take care of our environment!)

> Relatively few well-conducted studies have focused on the use of alternative therapies, such as herbs, to treat diabetes.

Free radicals are unstable molecules that can damage cells and tissues and can interfere with the immune system. (The immune system's job is to fight off infection and disease.) Free radicals are also implicated in heart disease because they favor plaque formation in the arteries, which can lead to atherosclerosis, also known as clogging of the arteries. Free radicals are partially to blame for cataract formation, arthritis, and even the effects of aging.

An *antioxidant* is a substance that prevents oxidative damage caused by free radicals. Antioxidants hold promise in preventing and treating diseases like cancer and heart disease. The benefits that antioxidants play in diabetes are still unclear. Certain nutrients have natural antioxidant qualities. Vitamin C, vitamin E, beta-carotene, and selenium all act as antioxidants to protect the body from oxidative damage. Fruits and vegetables are chock full of antioxidants. To reap the benefits, eat at least five servings per day from a combination of fruits and vegetables. (A serving is approximately 1 small piece, or ½ cup. The exchange lists in appendix A can be used for portioning.) Green tea also has antioxidant activity.

> Before you part with your money, it's important to be critical in your review of alternative therapies.

Tip: Eat at least five servings per day from a combination of fruits and vegetables.

Vitamin C

Besides acting as an antioxidant, vitamin C has many other useful functions. Among other things, it's important for wound healing and fighting infections. It also facilitates the absorption of iron; so if you take an iron supplement, eat a food rich in vitamin C at the same time and you'll absorb the iron better. Vitamin C is a water-soluble vitamin. Some of the vitamin C in foods is lost when the foods are cooked. Steaming or rapid cooking in a small amount of water can help to preserve the vitamin C content of foods. Raw foods contain the maximum amount of vitamin C.

When most people think of vitamin C, they think of orange juice. Sure, oranges are a great source of vitamin C, but so are many other foods.

The Following Foods Are All Rich in Vitamin C:

Bell peppers

Broccoli

Brussels sprouts

Cantaloupe

Cauliflower

Grapefruit

Greens (cabbage, spinach, collard, turnip, mustard, kale)

Honeydew melon

Kiwi fruit

Mango

Papaya

Potato

Strawberry

Sweet potato

Tangerine

Tomato

Watermelon

Vitamin C Requirements

Recommended Dietary Allowance (RDA) for Vitamin C (in milligrams per day)

Adult women: 75

Pregnant women: 85

Lactating women: 120

Adult men: 90

The Tolerable Upper Intake Level (UL) for all adults is set at 2,000 milligrams per day.

Caution: Supplementation with vitamin C at the upper intake levels may cause upset stomach and diarrhea.

Vitamin E "Tocopherol"

Vitamin E is a fat-soluble vitamin. This vitamin is not lost by most cooking methods, except the high heat of deep-frying. The main function of vitamin E is to serve as an antioxidant. Fruits, vegetables, and grains supply some vitamin E, but salad oils and margarine supply the most. Vitamin E deficiency is very rare.

The Following Foods Are All Rich in Vitamin E:

Almonds

Apricots

Avocado

Corn oil

Green leafy vegetables

Mangos

Margarine

Mayonnaise

Milk

Peanuts

Peas

Salmon

Safflower oil

Soybean oil

Sunflower oil

Wheat germ

Tip: As you probably noticed, many foods rich in vitamin E happen to be high in fat. If you're trying to lose weight, you shouldn't eat more fat; instead you may choose to supplement vitamin E.

Vitamin E "Tocopherol" Requirements

Recommended Dietary Allowance (RDA) for Vitamin E (in milligrams per day)

Adult women: 15

Pregnant women: 15

Lactating women: 19

Adult men: 15

The Tolerable Upper Intake Level (UL) for all adults is set at 1,000 milligrams per day.

Tip: Vitamin E is sometimes measured in international units. To convert from milligrams (mg) to international units (IU), multiply by 1.5. For example: 15 mg = 22 IU, and 19 mg = 28 IU.

> A pharmacist can advise you on interactions the herbal preparation could have with other medications that you take.

Beta-Carotene

Beta-carotene is in the class of nutrients known as carotenoids. There are more than 600 types of carotenoids. Carotenoids, abundant in fruits and vegetables, have antioxidant properties. People who consume diets that are high in fruits and vegetables appear to have less risk for developing certain diseases, including cancer, stroke, and heart disease. Although eating fruits and vegetables has been shown to have health benefits, isolating individual carotenoids and taking them in pill form has not always shown clear-cut health benefits. Supplementation study results range from positive effects to negative health outcomes. Supplementation of carotenoids is not a replacement for eating whole foods.

Beta-carotene's other important role is that it's converted to vitamin A in the body. Vitamin A is necessary for vision, healthy skin, fighting infections, reproduction, and normal growth and development. Beta-carotene is a fat-soluble nutrient. Cooking doesn't destroy it. A very large intake of dietary carotenoids can produce a yellowing of the skin, as avid drinkers of carrot juice can attest!

The Following Foods Are All Rich in Beta-Carotene:

Apricots

Asparagus

Broccoli

Cantaloupe

Carrots

Leafy greens (lettuce and all cooked greens)

Mango

Peach

Pink grapefruit

Pumpkin

Red bell peppers

Sweet potato

Tomato

Winter squashes

If you do decide to try an herbal supplement, discuss it with your health-care provider.

Beta-Carotene Requirements

No RDAs have been set for beta-carotene. Until more supplementation studies are done to prove safety, carotenoids should be obtained from a healthful intake of fruits and vegetables and not from a pill, *unless under medical supervision.*

Selenium

Selenium is a trace mineral. Selenium works in partnership with vitamin E to prevent oxidative damage. The selenium content of food varies according to where it was grown, as soil and water selenium concentrations vary. Selenium deficiency in the United States is very rare.

The Following Foods Are All Rich in Selenium:

Brazil nuts

Bread

Cereal

Eggs

Fish

Liver

Meats

Pinto beans

Poultry

Shellfish

Soybeans

Sunflower seeds

Tofu

Wheat germ

Whole grains

Selenium Requirements

Recommended Dietary Allowance (RDA) for Selenium (in micrograms per day)

Adult women: 55

Pregnant women: 60

Lactating women: 70

Adult men: 55

The Tolerable Upper Intake Level (UL) for all adults is set at 400 micrograms per day.

Final Tip

If you aren't sure whether you should take a vitamin or mineral supplement, you may want to contact a registered dietitian. A registered dietitian can evaluate your diet and your medical history to determine if a supplement could be beneficial. To find a registered dietitian in your area, call 1-800-366-1655.

CHAPTER 21

Eat Well, Be Well

❦

In This Chapter

- Reducing fat intake
- Reducing cholesterol intake
- Reducing sodium intake
- Reducing sugar intake
- Strategies for special occasions and holidays

This chapter provides tips on implementing a healthful diet. Whether shopping and cooking for yourself, grabbing something on the run, or sitting down to a fine dining experience at a favorite restaurant, what you eat directly affects your health and well-being.

Think of how many meals we consume in a lifetime. Not only is eating necessary, it's one of life's pleasures. We share memories over meals. We celebrate holidays and birthdays over meals. We can eat, drink, and be merry and still eat foods that promote health. So choose well, eat well, and be well.

Reducing Fat Intake
Shopping Lowfat

Eating healthfully starts with buying healthful foods, low in fat. That way, when hunger draws you into your kitchen and you open the cupboard or refrigerator, they'll be well stocked with appropriate food choices. It's easy to rush out to a store and buy the same old products, over and over. We're creatures of habit. But it's never too late to make positive changes. Take yourself on a field trip to your local grocery store. Plan on spending some time. Take a notepad and a pen and tour the aisles in search of healthful food choices. Take notes. Ask the store clerks.

Some Words of Advice

First, don't go shopping when you're hungry. It's too easy to buy the wrong things. A hungry stomach has too much influence over what goes into your cart! Shopping when you're tired or in a hurry can also lead to the wrong selections.

Second, read labels. Look at the ingredient list to see if there are added fats. Look at the total grams of fat: Three grams of fat per single serving means lowfat, and 3 grams of fat per ounce indicates a lowfat meat or cheese selection. For entrées, the limit should be 10 grams of fat per entrée. Make sure to buy products low in saturated fats.

> Not only is eating necessary, it's one of life's pleasures. . . . We can eat, drink, and be merry and still eat foods that promote health.

Lowfat Shopping List
Fruits and Vegetables

- Choose plenty of fresh produce.
- All fruits and vegetables are fat-free (except for avocados, olives, and coconuts).
- Choose fresh, frozen, or canned fruits (canned in their own juice or water, not syrup).
- Choose fresh, frozen, or canned vegetables that have not been processed with fats or sauces.

Grains and Legumes

- Choose unprocessed whole grains such as brown rice, wild rice, bulgar, kasha, couscous, millet, quinoa, barley, and rye.

- Choose pasta, especially whole grain varieties.

- Choose whole grain breads and rolls.

- Choose pita bread, French bread, or sourdough bread.

- Choose English muffins.

- Choose corn tortillas or lowfat flour tortillas.

- Choose oatmeal, grits, or other cooked cereals.

- Choose dried cereals without nuts, coconut, or added oils.

- Choose dried beans (or canned) such as garbanzo, kidney, northern, black, red, or pinto.

- Choose split peas and lentils.

- Choose fat-free canned refried beans.

Limit or avoid: Donuts, Danish, croissants, biscuits, muffins, waffles, pancakes, foccacia, fried chow mein noodles, cornbread, high-fat crackers, buttered popcorn, cheese crackers, peanut butter crackers, granola, croutons, refried beans with added lard or oils, and instant or processed grain or noodle dishes that have added fats.

Protein Foods

- Choose fresh fish or frozen fish without batters or sauces.

- Choose tuna packed in water.

- Choose poultry such as chicken, turkey, or Cornish hens. Skinless white meat is the lowest in fat.

- Choose ground turkey or extra-lean ground sirloin.

- Choose lean meats such as "loin" and "round" cuts. Do the visual check. If you see white marbling of fat, steer clear.

- Choose 98 percent fat-free hot dogs or lunch meats.

- Choose vegetarian protein sources. Try tofu, tempeh, seitan, and texturized vegetable protein. Look for vegi-burgers, tofu hot dogs, and vegetarian breakfast links.

- 3 grams of fat per ounce designates a lowfat meat choice.

298 EAT WELL, BE WELL

Limit or avoid: Bacon, regular hot dogs or lunch meats, sausage, ribs, corned beef, keilbasa, salami, breaded/fried chicken or fish, and fatty cuts of meat.

Dairy Section

- Choose nonfat or lowfat milk.
- Choose nonfat dry milk powder.
- Choose evaporated skim milk.
- Choose nonfat Lactaid milk if you're lactose intolerant.
- Choose nonfat, calcium-fortified soy milk or rice milk.
- Choose nonfat or lowfat yogurt.
- Choose nonfat or lowfat cottage cheese.
- Choose nonfat or lowfat sour cream.
- Choose nonfat or lowfat cream cheese or Neufchatel.
- Choose nonfat or lowfat cheese.
- Choose nonfat American cheese.
- 3 grams of fat per ounce designates a lowfat cheese or milk choice.

Limit or avoid: Whole milk, whole milk yogurt, whole milk cottage cheese, half-and-half, cream cheese, sour cream, cream, whipping cream, and all regular varieties of cheese.

Fats

- Choose lowfat margarine.
- Choose nonfat or lowfat mayonnaise.
- Choose nonfat or lowfat salad dressings.
- Choose spray oil or nonfat cooking sprays.

Limit or avoid: Butter, margarine, shortening, lard, mayonnaise, high-fat salad dressings, and excessive use of added oils, high-fat spreads, or sauces.

Tip: Limit all fats. When you do use fat, use the heart-healthier oils whenever possible (canola oil, olive oil, peanut oil).

Snacks

- Choose lowfat crackers.
- Choose Melba toast, bread sticks, or matzoh.
- Choose graham crackers.
- Choose pretzels.
- Choose air-popped popcorn.
- Choose microwaved "light" popcorn.
- Choose rice cakes.
- Choose baked potato chips or baked corn chips.
- Snack on fresh vegetables or a piece of fruit.
- Choose fat-free fudgesicles or popsicles (sugar-free versions available).
- Choose nonfat pudding or gelatin (sugar-free versions available).
- Choose frozen yogurt or reduced-fat ice cream (limit portion size).
- Choose angel food cake.

Eating healthfully starts with buying healthful foods, low in fat. That way, when hunger draws you into your kitchen and you open the cupboard or refrigerator, they'll be well stocked with appropriate food choices.

Limit or avoid: Nuts, seeds, fried items, pork rinds, regular chips, granola bars, candy bars, full-fat ice creams, cookies, pies, cakes, and trail mix.

Cooking Lowfat

Lowfat cooking methods help to keep the calories down. There are plenty of ways to prepare food without adding fat, so you should try to cook lowfat most of the time. If you have a favorite food that must be fried, limit the frequency and the portion size. In other words, if you absolutely love fried chicken, then it's probably important to you to include it once in a while. But don't go overboard! You'll probably stick to a healthful diet better if you don't feel as if you have to give everything up, all of the time.

Lowfat Cooking Methods

- Bake: in the oven.
- Broil: under the broiler; use a rack so the fat drips away from the meat.
- Boil: in water or broth.
- Braise: add liquid and bake in the oven.
- Blacken: sear in a very hot, dry pan.
- Poach: submerse in liquid and simmer on stovetop or heat in oven.
- Steam: in a steaming basket with a small amount of water below the basket.
- Roast: on a rack in the oven.
- Grill or barbecue: on the outdoor barbecue.
- Microwave: in the microwave oven, dry or with a little added liquid.
- Simmer: in broth instead of oil.
- Use a non-stick pan, with non-stick vegetable oil spray.
- Lightly sauté: with a teaspoon of oil in a hot pan or wok.
- Cook with wine; the alcohol will cook out and the flavor will stay.
- Don't add fats after cooking!
- Flavor foods with herbs and seasonings, flavored vinegar, fat-free chicken broth or vegetable broth, lemon, ginger, salsa, fat-free gravy, fat-free marinades, and fat-free dressings.

Avoid High-Fat Cooking Methods

Don't deep-fry foods; don't pan-fry in excessive amounts of oil; and don't use added fats, fatty sauces, or full-fat cheeses in preparing foods.

Buy a lowfat cookbook, or check one out from the library. You can also modify some of your favorite recipes. Try the tips in table 21.1 to decrease the fat content of the recipe.

Tabel 21.1   Recipe Modification Tips to Reduce Fat Content

Instead of this . . .	Try this more healthful alternative
Whole Milk	Nonfat Milk, Lowfat Milk
Whipped Cream	Nonfat Whipped Topping
Sour Cream	Nonfat/Lowfat Sour Cream, Nonfat Plain Yogurt
Regular Cheese	Reduced-Fat Cheese
Regular Cottage Cheese	Nonfat Cottage Cheese
Cream Cheese	Nonfat or Light Cream Cheese or Neufchatel
Butter and Stick Margarine	Reduced-Fat Margarine
Ice Cream	Nonfat Ice Cream, Frozen Yogurt
Cream or Half & Half	Nonfat Creamer or Evaporated Skim Milk
Bacon	Canadian Bacon or Ham
Sausage	Turkey Sausage or Veggie Soy Links
Hot Dogs	Reduced-Fat Hot Dogs, Soy/Tofu Hot Dogs
Bologna or Salami	Lowfat Bologna, Tofu Bologna
Red Meat Marbled with Fat	Lean Cuts: Sirloin, Tenderloin, Round, Flank
Ribs	Lean Cuts of Meat, Trimmed of Fat
Poultry with Skin	Skinless Poultry
Fried Meats	Grilled, Poached, Baked, Broiled, BBQ . . .
Ham Hocks or Salt Pork	Smoked Turkey or Lean Ham
High-Fat TV Dinners	TV Dinners with Less Than 10 Grams of Fat
Mayonnaise	Fat-Free or Lowfat Mayonnaise

Additional modifications

- You can also try reducing the amount of fat used. Reduce by one-quarter to one-third. Some recipes still work when the fat is cut by half.

- Refrigerate broths obtained from cooked meats. Remove the solid fat that forms at the top. Then make your soups or gravies from the de-fatted broth.

- Use a gravy skimmer to separate oil from the gravy.

Baking lowfat

- Replace the fat in quick breads, cakes, muffins, and brownies with pureed fruits like applesauce, prune puree, or mashed bananas. The result will be a lowfat, yet moist, product.

- Make single crust pies.

- Omit the nuts.

> Don't go shopping when you're hungry. It's too easy to buy the wrong things.

Lowfat Restaurant Tips

It's nice to go out to eat. Let someone else do all the work! But don't think of going out to eat as a reason to forget about healthful eating. Make wise menu selections. If you need more information to make the right choice, ask the waiter or chef for details about the menu items.

The portion that the restaurant serves isn't necessarily the best portion for your needs. If it looks too large, ask for a container and put some away before you dig in. Save it for lunch the next day. Or share an entrée with a friend and order additional salad and vegetables to complete the meal. Remember, you don't have to be a member of the clean plate club.

If you have a high-fat favorite food, try getting one order and sharing it with your dinner party. Ordering a dessert with "four forks" is another way to control your portion.

Menu Options

Appetizers to Choose

- Broth-based soups, tomato-based soups, or bean soups

- Green salad with dressing on the side (Ask for reduced-fat salad dressings or oil and vinegar. Or bring a small, leak-proof bottle of your own lowfat salad dressing.)

- Three bean salad

- Unbuttered bread or dinner rolls

- Shrimp or crab cocktail with cocktail sauce (Shrimp is relatively high in cholesterol but very low in saturated fat.)

Appetizers to Limit or Avoid

- Creamed soup

- Fatty salad dressings

- Mayonnaise-based salads such as cole slaw or potato salad

- Anything fried (chips, egg rolls, potato skins, fried zucchini, French fries, onion rings)

- Guacamole

- Buttered bread or rolls

- Croissants, biscuits, foccacia breads

Salad Bar Items to Choose

- Lettuce, spinach, greens, tomatoes, vegetables

- Legumes/beans

- Plain tuna without mayonnaise

- Sliced, skinless chicken or turkey

- Fresh fruit

- Cottage cheese

- Reduced-fat salad dressing
- Vinegar and a little oil

Salad Bar Items to Limit or Avoid

- Cheese
- Chopped egg
- Mayonnaise-based salads such as cole slaw, potato salad, or macaroni salad
- Fatty meats such as salami and crumbled bacon
- Olives and avocados (Although these are the heart-healthy type of fat, they're high in fat.)
- Croutons, chow mein noodles, nuts, sunflower seeds
- High-fat salad dressings such as blue cheese, ranch, Thousand Island

Entrées to Choose

- Meats, chicken, or fish cooked by lowfat methods
- Stir-fried vegetable dishes
- Sliced chicken, turkey, or ham sandwich made with mustard, not mayo
- Pasta primavera with tomato sauce or wine sauce
- Linguini with clams or mussels (in tomato sauce)
- Bean taco made with soft-shell corn tortillas, lettuce, tomato, and salsa
- Bean and chicken burrito with lettuce, tomato, salsa
- Broth-based noodle soups such as udon
- Tabbouleh and pita bread
- Tandoori chicken or fish, dal (lentils), biryani (rice), chapatis or nan (bread)

- Vegetable and grain mixtures

- Tofu, rice, and vegetables

- Ratatouille or other vegetable medleys

- Seafood soups such as bouillabaisse

- Ask your waiter for lowfat menu ideas specific to the restaurant that you visit.

Entrées to Limit or Avoid

- Anything deep fried or pan fried, cream sauce, mayonnaise-based tuna or egg salad sandwiches, pastrami, salami, sausages, lunch meat, dishes with cheese as a main ingredient, guacamole and sour cream toppings, coconut milk–based curries, duck, quiche, breaded items, lasagna, pesto sauce, Alfredo sauce, hollandaise sauce, béarnaise sauce, bechamel sauce, battered items, tempura, spanokopita or other items made with phyllo dough, au gratin, fritters, pot pies, chimichangas, chorizo, and dishes made with a roux sauce such as etouffee.

> Read labels. Look at the ingredient list to see if there are added fats.

- If in doubt about fat content, ask your waiter or the chef. Sometimes the restaurant will modify a menu item to make it lower in fat for you. It doesn't hurt to ask.

Side Dishes to Choose

- Baked potato topped with plain yogurt or cottage cheese

- Mashed potatoes (little or no gravy)

- Rice pilaf

- Steamed rice

- Pasta salad with vegetables (not mayonnaise-based)

- Tabouli or other grain-based salad

- Salads (not mayonnaise-based)
- Vegetables (raw, steamed, or lightly sautéed)

Side Dishes to Limit or Avoid

- Cole slaw, potato salad, French fries, onion rings, fried zucchini, potato skins, fried rice, and anything else that is fried

Desserts to Choose

- Fresh berries or melon
- Mixed fruit cup
- Small serving of frozen yogurt or ice milk (not ice cream)
- Angel food cake
- (I wish the list were longer too. If you choose to get something higher in calories, split it with your dinner partner.)

Desserts to Limit or Avoid

- Ice cream, custards, fried bananas, cakes, cookies, pies, pastries, anything with the word *decadence* in the title, or anything else that looks too good to be true!

Lowfat on the Go

I'm still waiting for someone to make a fast-food restaurant that serves only healthful choices. Boy, is it tough taking a road trip and finding that the only food options near the freeway are fast-food restaurants. I'd like to see more fast-food restaurants offer salad bars, vegi-burgers, and fresh fruit. How about we all ask or write to the giant corporations and request something tasty and low in fat and sodium?

Try to cook lowfat most of the time. If you have a favorite food that must be fried, limit the frequency and the portion size.

Until that day, use caution in what you order at fast-food restaurants. Ask for the nutrition facts brochure that lists the calorie and fat content of the menu items. Pick accordingly. Some restaurants post the menu information on the wall. I applaud them. Thanks.

Here are a few tips to get you in and out with the best bets.

Items to Choose in a Fast-Food Restaurant

- Plain burger with choice of ketchup, mustard, lettuce, tomato, onion, and pickle slice

- Grilled chicken sandwich (not breaded or fried)

- Grilled fish if they have it (not the breaded or fried fish sandwich, which has more fat than a burger)

- Chicken fajitas

- English muffin with Canadian bacon if desired

- Plain bagel with nonfat cream cheese

- Side salad with lowfat salad dressing (not the chef salad with fatty meat or cheese)

- Chicken salad with lowfat salad dressing

- Baked potato with choice of cottage cheese, vegetables, salsa, and lowfat sour cream

- Mashed potatoes

- *Share* a small bag of fries if you must

- Burrito with choice of beans, rice, chicken, lettuce, tomato, and salsa

- Soft taco (skip the sour cream, guacamole, and cheese)

- Roasted or rotisserie chicken; take off the skin

- Corn on the cob

- Steamed rice

- Chicken fajita pita

- Small-sized items, or the "kids meal"

- Baked beans

- Hot or cold cereals

- Frozen yogurt, lowfat ice cream cone, fruit

- Diet drinks, lowfat milk, coffee, tea, unsweetened iced tea

- There may be other appropriate items to choose that I haven't mentioned. Review nutrition facts brochures where available.

Items to Limit or Avoid at Fast-Food Restaurants

Double burgers, super-sized items, fried fish, breaded fish or chicken sandwiches, French fries, curly fries, hash browns, fried rice, egg rolls, stuffed and fried jalapenos, breaded chicken nuggets, breaded fried shrimp, nachos, pizza, potato salad, cole slaw, fried chicken, hot wings, onion rings, breakfast sandwiches, sausage and bacon, croissants, biscuits, cornbread, Danish, pastries, hot dogs, pies, cookies, ice cream, regular sodas, milk shakes, whole milk, tartar sauce, mayonnaise, regular salad dressings, guacamole, cheese, cream cheese, and anything else they're frying up that day. (I'm sure I left some things out.)

Try not to rely on fast-food restaurants too often. Try packing a healthful lunch to take with you. You'll have a lot more control over what you eat.

Airline Meals

Airlines offer special meals. You can order a variety of meals, including heart-healthy, diabetes-friendly, lowfat, low sodium, and vegetarian meals. Inquire about the options next time you book a flight. Special meals must be ordered before the day of your flight to allow for preparation and delivery.

Reducing Cholesterol Intake

Plant foods don't have any cholesterol, which means that fruits, vegetables, and grains are all cholesterol-free. Cholesterol is found only in animal products. The foods that are particularly high in cholesterol include egg yolks, organ meats, shrimp, squid, and large portions of meat or poultry.

Strategies for Cutting Down on Dietary Cholesterol Intake

- Instead of one egg, try two egg whites, or ¼ cup egg substitute.

- Instead of organ meats, choose lean cuts of meat, trimmed of fat.

- Limit intake of shrimp and squid to occasional use. Choose fresh fish instead.

- Limit your meat and poultry portions to the size of the palm of your hand.

- Instead of meat-based main dishes, try more vegetarian main dishes.

Cholesterol is also produced within your own body, by your liver. Saturated fats (animal fats and solid fats) can cause your body to produce more cholesterol. In fact, cutting back on saturated fat is even more important than reducing dietary cholesterol intake. Choose nonfat and lowfat dairy products. Limit the use of solid fats such as shortening, margarine, butter, coconut oil, palm oil, or lard. Replace those artery-clogging fats with heart-healthier liquid oils. The calories are about the same when it comes to your weight, but it's an improvement in the type of fat that you use when considering heart health.

> The portion that the restaurant serves isn't necessarily the best portion for your needs. If it looks too large, ask for a container and put some away before you dig in.

For more information on cholesterol and fats, see chapter 11 on cardiac health.

Reducing Sodium Intake

Did you know that salt is a preservative? In the past, before refrigeration, curing foods helped ensure that they didn't spoil. Salt is still added to many foods to improve shelf life. Many packaged and processed foods are high in salt.

Sodium is another word for salt. Actually, table salt is made of sodium and chloride. The words *salt* and *sodium* are often used interchangeably.

If you have high blood pressure or take medications to control blood pressure, you may want to decrease your sodium intake. As you cut back on your salt intake, your taste buds will adjust.

Shopping for Low-Sodium Foods

Fresh is the best. When foods are bought in their natural, unprocessed state, they're low in sodium. When it comes to packaged foods, read food labels to choose appropriately.

Ranking Sodium

Sodium-free is less than 5 mg per serving.

Very low sodium is less than 35 mg per serving.

Low sodium is less than 140 mg per serving.

Moderate sodium is between 140 and 400 mg per serving.

High sodium is over 400 mg per serving.

Entrées should have less than 800 mg sodium per entrée.

Daily sodium intake should be 2,400 mg or less.

Lower-Sodium Shopping List
Fruits and Vegetables

- Choose plenty of fresh produce.
- All fresh fruits and vegetables are relatively sodium-free.
- Choose frozen or canned vegetables with no added salt.
- Choose carrot juice or fresh blended vegetable juices.
- Choose low-sodium tomato juice or low-sodium V-8.

- Choose low-sodium tomato sauce.
- Choose tomato paste.

Limit or avoid: Pickled vegetables, pickles, olives, sauerkraut, kim chi, frozen or canned vegetables with added salt, canned tomato sauce, canned tomato juice, and V-8.

Soups

- Choose homemade soups or broths without added salts.
- Choose low-sodium canned soups and broths.
- Choose low-sodium dehydrated soup mixes.

Limit or avoid: All regular canned soups, bouillon cubes, broth, cup of soup, cup of noodles, ramen noodles, and dehydrated soup mixes.

Grains and Legumes

- Choose unprocessed whole grains such as brown rice, wild rice, bulgar, kasha, couscous, millet, quinoa, barley, and rye.
- Choose unprocessed pasta, spaghetti, noodles, and macaroni.
- Choose breads, bagels, and rolls without salted tops.
- Choose flour or corn tortillas.
- Choose dried beans, split peas, and lentils and cook them yourself.
- Rinse canned beans under running water to remove some of the salt.
- Choose unseasoned bread crumbs or stuffing mix.
- Choose lower-sodium cereals (read labels).

Limit or avoid: Instant pasta and potato dishes, instant seasoned rice mixes, cup of noodles, ramen noodles, macaroni and cheese mix, canned beans with salt added, bread crumb coating mixes, croutons, waffle or pancake mixes, and seasoned stuffing mix. Many breakfast cereals have significant amounts of sodium (especially flake cereals), so read the food labels.

Protein Foods

- Choose fresh or frozen fish, poultry, or meats (without batters or sauces).

- Choose eggs or egg substitutes.

- Choose low-sodium canned fish.

- Choose water-packed canned chicken.

Limit or avoid: Salted and cured meats such as bacon, jerky, hot dogs, lunch meats, sausage, corned beef, keilbasa, salami, Spam, sardines, caviar, and anchovies.

Dairy Section

- Choose milk and yogurt

- Choose low-sodium cheeses, low-sodium cottage cheese, ricotta cheese, and mozzarella cheese.

Limit or avoid: Buttermilk, regular cheeses, processed cheese spread, and regular cottage cheese.

Fats

- Choose unsalted butter and margarine, vegetable oils, and low-sodium salad dressings.

- Keep in mind that these are all still high in fat!

Limit or avoid: Salted butter and margarine and some regular salad dressings (read labels).

Snacks

- Choose unsalted versions of crackers, bread sticks, pretzels, rice cakes, popcorn, potato chips, and corn chips.

- Choose unsalted nuts and seeds (caution: they're still high in fat).

- Snack on fresh vegetables or a piece of fruit.

Limit or avoid: Pork rinds and cheese curls, salted versions of nuts, seeds, crackers, bread sticks, pretzels, popcorn, and chips. Look out for cakes and instant puddings; they can be sources of hidden sodium.

Low-Sodium Cooking

The best way to reduce the sodium in cooking at home is to get rid of the salt shaker! Don't add salt to the cooking water for rice or pasta. Don't salt foods while you cook, and don't salt foods at the table. One single teaspoon of salt has over 2,300 mg of sodium.

You aren't doing yourself a favor by using seasoning salt, onion salt, garlic salt, or celery salt. They're all still salt. They're just flavored salts.

The good news is that you can season foods plenty of ways without using salt. You might just have to experiment a little. Break away from the old habits and try some new flavors. Try using a cookbook that boasts low sodium.

Seasoning Low-Sodium

Choose These Herbs and Spices

Allspice, anise, basil, bay, capsicum, caraway, cardamom, celery seed, chervil, chili powder, chives, cilantro, cinnamon, cloves, coriander, cumin, curry, dill, fennel seed, fenugreek seed, garlic powder, ginger, mace, marjoram, mint, ground mustard, nutmeg, onion powder, oregano, paprika, parsley, black pepper, white pepper, red pepper, poppy seeds, poultry seasoning, rosemary, saffron, sage, savory, tarragon, thyme, and turmeric.

More Choices

- Flavored extracts such as vanilla, almond, or coconut extract
- Seasoned vinegars
- Sesame oil and toasted sesame oil

- Red onions, green onions, shallots, leeks
- Fresh garlic
- Fresh ginger root
- Lemon and lime juices
- Fresh chili peppers
- Tabasco
- Horseradish
- Mustard and ketchup (limit to 1–2 teaspoons, as large amounts will add up sodium)
- Commercial herb blends like Mrs. Dash
- Cooking with wine (the alcohol cooks out)
- Fresh-cut tomato salsa (prepared without added salt)
- Low-sodium broth
- Low-sodium salad dressings
- Low-sodium sauces

Limit or avoid: Salt, soy sauce, steak sauce, teriyaki sauce, A-1 sauce, hollandaise sauce, béarnaise sauce, cocktail sauce, canned spaghetti sauce unless it is low sodium, tomato sauce, canned salsa, pickle relish, commercial canned sauces, or sauce mixes.

A Word About Salt Substitutes

- First of all, light salt and light soy sauce still have a lot of sodium.
- Some of the other salt substitutes are made from potassium. They don't have any sodium. If you have kidney problems or take blood pressure medications, then check with your doctor before using potassium-based salt substitutes. The extra potassium could cause blood potassium levels to rise too much. Certainly, if you're on a low-potassium diet, you should avoid potassium-based salt substitutes.

Low-Sodium Restaurant Tips

- Take the tips contained in the previous sections on shopping and cooking low in sodium, and apply the same principle to ordering low-sodium restaurant meals.

- Ask the waiter or chef for suggestions.

- Ask if it's possible to have your foods prepared without added salt.

- Don't salt your foods at the table.

- Order sauces and salad dressings on the side, and use sparingly.

- Choose salad instead of soup.

- Use limited amounts of condiments.

- Skip the pickles and pickle relish.

- Skip the soy sauce.

- Limit trips to fast-food restaurants because many menu items are high in sodium. (Look at fast-food nutrition facts provided by the restaurant and choose the best possible options.)

Reducing Sugar Intake

Although it's okay for people with diabetes to consume some sugar, too much sugar can have a negative impact on the blood sugar and the weight. Concentrated sweets can provide excessive amounts of calories, and, generally speaking, the calories are devoid of nutrition. It's not a bad idea for all of us to watch our sugar intake.

Be sure to read food labels for the total carbohydrate content and the calories, not just sugar grams. Just because something is sugar-free doesn't mean it's free of carbohydrate or even low in calories.

> Desserts to limit or avoid: anything with the word *decadence* in the title, or anything else that looks too good to be true!

Low-Sugar Products

- Sugar substitutes
- All diet soft drinks, including sugar-free ice tea, sugar-free Kool Aid, Crystal Light
- All diet sodas
- Unsweetened, or diet iced tea
- Unsweetened, flavored mineral waters
- Sugar-free gelatin
- No-sugar-added puddings
- No-sugar-added hot cocoa mix
- Aspartame-sweetened yogurts
- Reduced-sugar ice creams and frozen yogurts
- No-sugar-added ice cream bars and fudge pops
- Sugar-free popsicles
- No-sugar-added jams and jellies
- Diet pancake syrup
- Sugar-free gum
- Sugar-free breath mints

See chapter 16 on sugars and sweeteners for tips on using artificial sweeteners in place of sugar in cooking and baking.

Strategies for Special Occasions and Holidays

Festivities, parties, and holidays are often celebrated by preparing and partaking of special meals and tasty treats. It can be challenging to stay in control of what and how much you eat! There are strategies for staying on track. When possible, improve recipes by reducing fat, cholesterol, sodium, and sugar. For items that are too tempting to forgo, keep the portion small. Baking for the holidays is fine. Allow yourself a taste or a small portion, and then be prompt about giving the rest away as gifts. Consider making ornaments or other craft items instead of sweet treats.

Tips for Special Occasions

- Eat slowly. Enjoy the get-together. Focus on the friends and family. Take the focus off the food.

- Have a healthful snack to curb your appetite before the celebration begins.

- You'll have more control if you don't arrive at a party hungry.

- Plan ahead. Think about how you will handle the special occasion. Choose specific dietary behaviors that you plan to adhere to. For example, you may decide that you'll avoid all fried items or limit yourself to a specific portion size.

- Make and bring a healthful dish to ensure that at least one nutritious choice will be available.

- Choose larger portions of the low-calorie items and smaller portions of the higher-calorie items.

- Fresh vegetables are always a good choice.

- Choose calorie-free beverages.

- Don't eat out of presumed obligation. Politely refuse when you really don't want something.

- Eat until you are satisfied (not stuffed). Don't overeat.

- Go for a walk after the meal.

- If you get carried away, try to get back on track the next day. Don't give up.

Thanksgiving Menu Modifications

- Choose white meat turkey and don't eat the skin.

- Don't add butter or nuts to the stuffing mix.

- Cook the stuffing in the oven, not in the bird. It's much lower in fat.

- Instead of the drippings from the turkey, use fat-free turkey or chicken broth to make the gravy. Boil the broth. Add seasonings. Stir in a mixture of cornstarch or flour that has been mixed smoothly into water. Simmer.

- Make your own stock from boiling the carcass. After refrigeration, remove the fat that has solidified on top. Use the de-fatted broth to make soup with the leftover turkey.

- Use nonfat milk or evaporated skim milk to make the mashed potatoes. Skip the butter or margarine.

- Instead of candied yams, bake sweet potatoes in their jackets until very soft. Scoop them out and mash.

- Serve fresh steamed green vegetables.

- Serve a festive mixed salad with lowfat salad dressing.

- Serve fresh warm dinner rolls and skip the butter.

- To make cranberry sauce, boil fresh cranberries in water. Add cinnamon, cloves, and ground ginger. Simmer to desired consistency. Remove from heat, then add artificial sweetener instead of sugar. (The artificial sweetener should be added after the cooking process, because high temperatures can alter the taste of some artificial sweeteners.)

- For pumpkin pies, use evaporated skim milk in place of half-and-half. Use egg substitute or egg whites in place of whole eggs. (One egg equals two egg whites or ¼ cup egg substitute.) Cut down on the sugar. Use lowfat whipped topping instead of real whipped cream.

Bon appétit!

Excerpts from
the Exchange Lists

∽

Things to Notice When Using the Exchange Lists

- Starches are measured after they are cooked.

- Breads, rolls, and bagels are all 15 grams of carbohydrate *per ounce*. A large bagel weighs about 4 ounces, which is equal to 60 grams of carbohydrate or 4 starch exchanges. A food scale can come in handy for weighing bread products.

- Fruits are weighed with the peelings and skins still on.

- Grapefruit juice has the same amount of carbohydrate as apple juice (15 grams per ½ cup). Tart-tasting fruits can have as much carbohydrate as sweet-tasting fruits. All juices are concentrated sources of carbohydrate.

- The milk list contains only milk and yogurt.

- Cheese, sour cream, half-and-half, cream, butter, and cream cheese do not contain carbohydrate so they are not grouped with the milk. When you milk a cow, what comes to the top of the pail? Cream. Cream is fat. If you whip cream long enough, it turns to butter. Butter is on the fat list. If you take the cream from the top of the milk pail and culture it, you get sour cream. Sour cream is fat, and so is cream cheese, and half-and-half. They all end up on the fat list.

- Regular cheeses are made from the protein and the fat from whole milk. The liquid carbohydrate (lactose) is removed when the cheese is made. Cheese ends up being high in protein and fat, so it's on the high-fat meat list.

- Starchy vegetables like potato, corn, peas, yam, and sweet potato are listed on the starch list, not the vegetable list. They each contain about 15 grams of carbohydrate per ½ cup.

- Three portions of nonstarchy vegetables (5 grams carbohydrate each) are the same amount of carbohydrate as eating one portion of starch, fruit, or milk.

- Nonstarchy vegetables are low in calories. One portion of vegetables has only 25 calories. If you add one teaspoon of butter, you add an additional 45 calories. The butter topping has more calories than the vegetables.

- Three ounces of meat is roughly the size of a deck of cards.

- High-fat meats have almost twice as many calories as lean meats. For example, 3 ounces of lean meat has 165 calories (55 calories per ounce), and 3 ounces of high-fat meat has 300 calories (100 calories per ounce). The type of meat that you select can have a big impact on your weight and your heart.

- Everything on the fats list has the same amount of calories; therefore, eating 6 almonds has the same amount of calories as 1 teaspoon of butter. Watch out for nuts. The calories can add up if you sit down with an open can of nuts in front of the television!

- Even though all fats have the same calories, the monounsaturated fats are more healthful for your heart. Select olive oil, canola oil, peanut oil, avocados, olives, nuts, or seeds over solid fats or animal fats (butter, margarine, cream, sour cream, etc.).

Starch List

All Selections: 80 Calories, 15 g Carbohydrate, 3 g Protein, 0–1 g Fat	
Note: Items are measured after cooking.	
bread (white, wheat, rye, etc.)	1 slice (weighing 1 oz.)
bagel	1 oz. (note: a large bagel may weigh 4 oz.; a small bagel may be closer to 2 oz.)
roll	1 small (weighing 1 oz.)
hamburger bun or hot dog bun	½ bun
English muffin	½
pita bread	½ (6-inch diameter)
corn tortilla	1 small (6-inch diameter)
flour tortilla	1 small (6-inch diameter)
rice (white or brown)	⅓ cup
couscous	⅓ cup
noodles/pasta	½ cup
oats	½ cup
grits	½ cup
bulgur	½ cup
kasha	½ cup
beans (pinto, kidney, garbanzo, etc.)	½ cup
split peas, black-eyed peas	½ cup
lentils	½ cup
lima beans	⅔ cup
baked beans	⅓ cup
miso	3 tbsp.
potato	1 small baked or boiled (weighing 3 oz.)
potato, mashed	½ cup
corn	½ cup
corn on the cob	1 medium (weighing 5 oz.)
green peas	½ cup
yam	½ cup
sweet potato	½ cup

Starch List (continued)

All Selections: 80 Calories, 15 g Carbohydrate, 3 g Protein, 0–1 g Fat	
Note: Items are measured after cooking.	
plantain	½ cup
winter squash (acorn, butternut, etc.)	1 cup
pumpkin	1 cup
saltine crackers	6
graham crackers	3 small squares
popcorn	3 cups popped
rice cakes	2 (4-inch diameter)
flour	3 tbsp. dry
cornmeal	3 tbsp. dry
wheat germ	3 tbsp.
The following starches still have 15 grams of carbohydrate, but they are higher in fat (5 grams of fat per serving).	
biscuit	1 small (2½ inches in diameter)
chow mein noodles	½ cup
cornbread	1 small (2-inch cube, weighing 2 oz.)
croutons	1 cup
French fries	16–25 fries (weighing 3 oz.)
muffin	small (weighing 1½ oz.)
pancakes	2 small (each 4 inches in diameter)
taco shells	2 crisp (6-inch size)
waffle	1 small (4½ inch square)
stuffing	⅓ cup prepared

Fruit List

All Selections: 60 Calories, 15 g Carbohydrate, 0 g Protein, 0 g Fat	
Note: The weights listed in parentheses include the weight of the skin, core, seeds, and rind, so don't peel the fruit until after it has been weighed.	
apple	1 small (4 oz.)
applesauce	½ cup unsweetened
apricots	4 whole fresh (5½ oz.)
apricots	8 halves dried
apricots	½ cup canned
banana	1 small (4 oz.)
blackberries	¾ cup
blueberries	¾ cup
cantaloupe	1 cup cubes (11 oz.)
cherries	12 fresh (3 oz.)
dates	3
figs	2 medium, fresh (3½ oz.)
figs	1½ dried
fruit cocktail	½ cup
grapefruit	½ large (11 oz.)
grapefruit	¾ cup canned
grapes	17 small (3 oz.)
honeydew	1 cup cubed (10 oz.)
kiwi fruit	1 (3½ oz.)
mango	½ small (5½ oz.), or ½ cup
nectarine	1 small (5 oz.)
orange	1 small (6½ oz.)
papaya	½ fruit (8 oz.), 1 cup cubed
peach	1 medium (6 oz.)
peaches	½ cup canned
pear	½ large (4 oz.)
pears	½ cup canned
pineapple	¾ cup fresh

Fruit List (continued)

All Selections: 60 Calories, 15 g Carbohydrate, 0 g Protein, 0 g Fat	
Note: The weights listed in parentheses include the weight of the skin, core, seeds, and rind, so don't peel the fruit until after it has been weighed.	
pineapple	½ cup canned
plums	2 small (5 oz.)
prunes	3 dried
raisins	2 tbsp.
raspberries	1 cup
strawberries	1¼ cups
tangerines	2 small (8 oz.)
watermelon	1 slice (13½ oz.), or 1¼ cups
apple juice/cider	½ cup
cranberry juice cocktail	⅓ cup
grape juice	⅓ cup
grapefruit juice	½ cup
orange juice	½ cup
pineapple juice	½ cup
prune juice	⅓ cup

Milk List

Fat-Free/Lowfat Selections: 90 Calories, 12–15 g Carbohydrate, 8 g Protein, 0–3 g Fat	
fat-free milk	1 cup
½% or 1% milk	1 cup
fat-free or lowfat buttermilk	1 cup
fat-free powdered dry milk	⅓ cup dry
evaporated skim milk	½ cup
plain nonfat yogurt	¾ cup
nonfat aspartame-sweetened yogurt	1 cup
Reduced Fat Selections: 120 Calories, 12–15 g Carbohydrate, 8 g Protein, 5 g Fat	
2% milk	1 cup
reduced-fat yogurt	¾ cup
Whole Selections: 150 Calories, 12–15 g Carbohydrate, 8 g Protein, 8 g Fat	
whole milk	1 cup
kefir	1 cup
evaporated whole milk	½ cup
whole goat's milk	1 cup
whole milk yogurt	¾ cup

Other Carbohydrates List

Everything on the following list counts as approximately 15 grams of carbohydrate or 1 carbohydrate exchange. Because of the nature of this list, the calories, protein, and fat contents vary. Read labels when possible.

1 brownie (small, unfrosted, 2-inch square)

cake (unfrosted, 2-inch square)

3 small gingersnaps

5 vanilla wafers

2 small crème-filled sandwich cookies

½ cup ice cream

⅓ cup frozen yogurt (fat-free or lowfat)

½ cup no-sugar-added frozen yogurt

½ cup regular gelatin

½ cup no-sugar-added pudding

¼ cup regular pudding

1 granola bar

1 tablespoon sugar, honey, syrup, jam, or jelly

Vegetable List

All Selections: 25 Calories, 5 g Carbohydrate, 2 g Protein, 0 g Fat

Note: One exchange (portion) from the vegetable list is ½ cup cooked vegetables, 1 cup raw vegetables, or ½ cup vegetable juice.

Artichoke, asparagus, beets, broccoli, brussels sprouts, cabbage, carrots, cauliflower, celery, cucumber, eggplant, green beans, greens, kohlrabi, leeks, mushrooms, okra, onions, pea pods, peppers, radishes, salad greens, sauerkraut, spinach, summer squash, tomatoes, tomato sauce, tomato juice, turnips, water chestnuts, watercress, vegetable juice, and zucchini

Meat and Meat Substitutes List

Very Lean Selections: 35 Calories, 0 g Carbohydrate, 7 g Protein, 0–1 g Fat	
chicken	1 oz. (skinless white meat)
turkey	1 oz. (skinless white meat)
Cornish hens	1 oz. (skinless)
fish (most varieties)	1 oz.
shellfish	1 oz.
venison	1 oz.
pheasant	1 oz.
buffalo	1 oz.
ostrich	1 oz.
egg substitutes	1 oz.
egg whites	2
nonfat or lowfat cottage cheese	¼ cup
nonfat cheeses	1 oz. (label states 0–1 grams of fat per oz.)
Lean Selections: 55 Calories, 0 g Carbohydrate, 7 g Protein, 3 g Fat	
lean beef	1 oz. (sirloin, tenderloin, round, or flank)
lean pork	1 oz. (tenderloin, ham, or Canadian bacon)
lean lamb	1 oz. (roast, chop, or leg)
lean veal	1 oz. (lean chop or roast)
skinless dark meat poultry	1 oz.
white meat poultry with skin	1 oz.
oily fish	1 oz. (herring, salmon, or sardines)
reduced-fat cheeses	1 oz. (label states 3 grams of fat, or less, per oz.)
grated parmesan cheese	2 tbsp.
lunch meats	1 oz. (label states 3 grams of fat, or less, per oz.)

Meat and Meat Substitutes List (continued)

Medium-Fat Selections: 75 Calories, 0 g Carbohydrate, 7 g Protein, 5 g Fat	
medium-fat beef	1 oz. (ground beef, meatloaf, corned beef, short ribs, prime rib, prime grades of meat)
medium-fat pork	1 oz. (top loin, chop, cutlet, Boston butt)
medium-fat lamb	1 oz. (rib roast, ground)
veal	1 oz. (cutlet, ground, or cubed)
dark meat chicken with the skin	1 oz.
fried fish	1 oz.
feta or mozzarella cheese	1 oz.
ricotta cheese	2 oz.
reduced-fat cheese	1 oz. (label states 5 grams of fat per oz.)
egg	1
tofu	½ cup
tempeh	¼ cup
High-Fat Selections: 100 Calories, 0 g Carbohydrate, 7 g Protein, 8 g Fat	
pork sausage	1 oz.
pork spareribs	1 oz.
bologna, salami	1 oz.
knockwurst, bratwurst	1 oz.
hotdog	1
sausage	1 oz.
bacon	3 slices
all regular cheeses	1 oz. (cheddar, Jack, Swiss, American . . .)

Fat List

All Selections: 45 Calories, 0 g Carbohydrate, 0 g Protein, 5 g Fat	
Note: Nuts and seeds do contain some protein and a small amount of carbohydrate, but they are predominantly fat.	
butter	1 tsp.
margarine	1 tsp.
vegetable oil (all varieties)	1 tsp.
mayonnaise (regular)	1 tsp.
mayonnaise (reduced-fat)	1 tbsp.
salad dressing (regular)	1 tbsp.
salad dressing (reduced fat)	2 tbsp.
avocado	⅛
olives	8 large
almonds or cashews	6
peanuts	10
peanut butter	2 tsp.
pecans	4 halves
pumpkin seeds	1 tbsp.
sunflower seeds	1 tbsp.
sesame seeds	1 tbsp.
tahini paste	2 tsp.
walnuts	4 halves
half-and-half cream	2 tbsp.
sour cream (regular)	2 tbsp.
sour cream (reduced-fat)	3 tbsp.
cream cheese (regular)	1 tbsp.
cream cheese (reduced-fat)	2 tbsp.
shortening	1 tsp.
lard	1 tsp.
bacon	1 slice
chitterlings, boiled	2 tbsp.

Measurements and Conversions

❧

Blood Sugar

1 mmol/l = 18 mg/dl

Weight Measures

1 g	= 0.035 oz	= 0.001 kg	= 1,000 mg
1 mg	= 0.001 g	= 1,000 mcg	
28 g	= 1 oz		
16 oz	= 1 lb	= 454 g	= 0.454 kg
2.2 lb	= 1 kg	= 1,000 g	

Volume Measures

1 tsp	= ⅓ tbsp	= ⅙ fl oz	= 5 ml
3 tsp	= 1 tbsp	= ½ fl oz	= 15 ml
2 tbsp	= ⅛ cup	= 1 fl oz	= 30 ml
4 tbsp	= ¼ cup	= 2 fl oz	= 59 ml
5⅓ tbsp	= ⅓ cup	= 2⅔ fl oz	= 79 ml
8 tbsp	= ½ cup	= 4 fl oz	= 118 ml

10⅔ tbsp	= ⅔ cup	= 5⅓ fl oz	= 158 ml
12 tbsp	= ¾ cup	= 6 fl oz	= 177 ml
16 tbsp	= 1 cup	= 8 fl oz	= 240 ml
1 pint	= 2 cups	= .473 liter	= 473 ml
1 quart	= 2 pints	= .946 liter	= 946 ml
1 gallon	= 4 quarts	= 3.785 liter	= 3,785 ml
1 liter	= 1.057 quarts	= 34 fl oz	= 1,000 ml

(For simplification, some numbers have been rounded.)

Abbreviations

mmol/l = millimoles per liter

mg/dl = milligrams per deciliter

g = gram

mg = milligram

mcg = microgram

kg = kilogram

oz = ounce

lb = pound

tsp = teaspoon

tbsp = tablespoon

fl oz = fluid ounce

ml = milliliter

Important Contacts

∽

American Association of Diabetes Educators

1-800-338-3633
www.aadenet.org

American Diabetes Association

1-800-232-3472
www.diabetes.org
http://store.diabetes.org (for book list/ordering)

American Dietetic Association

1-800-877-1600
1-800-366-1655 (consumer nutrition hotline in English and Spanish)
www.eatright.org

American Heart Association

1-800-242-8721
www.americanheart.org

Canadian Diabetes Association

www.diabetes.ca

Centers for Disease Control and Prevention

1-877-232-3422

www.cdc.gov/diabetes

Children with Diabetes

1-513-755-0186

www.childrenwithdiabetes.com

Diabetes Wellness

1-800-941-4635

www.diabeteswellness.net

Food and Drug Administration

1-888-463-6332

www.fda.gov

Joslin Diabetes Center

1-617-732-2400

www.joslin.harvard.edu

Juvenile Diabetes Foundation International

1-800-223-1138

www.jdfcure.org

National Heart, Lung, and Blood Institute

www.nhlbi.nih.gov/index.html

National Institute of Diabetes & Digestive & Kidney Diseases

1-301-654-3327

www.niddk.nih.gov

National Institutes of Health

www.nih.gov

Rick Mendosa's Diabetes Directory

A complete listing of Web addresses for everything related to diabetes.
www.mendosa.com/diabetes.htm

Weight-Control Information Network

1-877-946-4627
www.niddk.nih.gov/health/nutrit/nutrit.htm

Index